Keto Diet Cookbook for Beginners

The Best Tasty Protein Recipes to Support your Weight Loss | Delicious Protein Recipes

Jane Leaner

Copyright – 2021 – **Jane Leaner**

All rights reserved.

The content contained within this book may not be reproduced, duplicated, or transmitted without direct written permission from the author or the publisher.
Under no circumstances will any blame or legal responsibility be held against the publisher, or author, for any damages, reparation, or monetary loss due to the information contained within this book. Either directly or indirectly.

Legal Notice:

This book is copyright protected. This book is only for personal use. You cannot amend, distribute, sell, use, quote, or paraphrase any part, or the content within this book, without the consent of the author or publisher.

Disclaimer Notice:

Please note the information contained within this document is for educational and entertainment purposes only. All effort has been executed to present accurate, up to date, and reliable, complete information. No warranties of any kind are declared or implied. Readers acknowledge that the author is not engaging in the rendering of legal, financial, medical, or professional advice. The content within this book has been derived from various sources. Please consult a licensed professional before attempting any techniques outlined in this book.

By reading this document, the reader agrees that under no circumstances is the author responsible for any losses, direct or indirect, which are incurred as a result of the use of the information contained within this document, including, but not limited to, - errors, omissions, or inaccuracies.

Table of Content

1. Avocado Taco Boats 7
2. Bacon Cheeseburger 10
3. Baked Beef Zucchini 13
4. Cheeseburger Pie 15
5. Chocolate Orange Bites 17
6. Cinnamon Bites 19
7. Cocoa Brownies 21
8. Coconut Fudge 24
9. Easy Vanilla Bombs 26
10. Mozzarella Sticks 28
11. Nutmeg Nougat 30
12. Personal Pizza Biscuit 31
13. Pesto Crackers 33
14. Sausage and Cheese Dip 35
15. Steak and Avocado Lettuce Wraps 37
16. Strawberry Cheesecake Minis 40
17. Sweet Almond Bites 41
18. Sweet Chai Bites 42
19. Beef and Mushrooms 45
20. Beef Stroganoff 47
21. Cayenne Rib Eye Steak 48
22. Cheesy Taco Bake 51
23. Chili Beef Jerky 52
24. Greek Beef Roast 54
25. Avocado Lime Shrimp Salad 56
26. Baked Cod Crusted with Herbs 57
27. Baked Tuna with Asparagus 59
28. Cajun Garlic Shrimp Noodle Bowl 61
29. Caribbean Steamed Fish 63
30. Coconut Salsa on Chipotle Fish Tacos 65
31. Crazy Saganaki Shrimp 68
32. Creamy Bacon-Fish Chowder 70
33. Crisped Coco-Shrimp with Mango Dip 72
34. Crispy Fish 75

35.	Cucumber-Basil Salsa on Halibut Pouches	76
36.	Curry Salmon with Mustard	78
37.	Dill Relish on White Sea Bass	79
38.	Dijon Mustard and Lime Marinated Shrimp	81
39.	Healthy Salmon	84
40.	Miso-Glazed Salmon	86
41.	Mussels Mariners	88
42.	Salmon with Vegetables	90
43.	Salmon Florentine	92
44.	Salmon Burgers	95
45.	Salmon Cakes	97
46.	Savory Cilantro Salmon	98
47.	Scampi Grilled Shrimp	101
48.	Seared Scallops	102
49.	Shrimp Broccoli	104
50.	Shrimp Chives Chipotle	106
51.	Shrimp Curry	108

1. Avocado Taco Boats

Preparation time: 5 minutes

Cooking time: 20 minutes

Servings: 4

Ingredients:
- 4 grape tomatoes
- 2 large avocados
- 1 lb. ground beef
- 4 tablespoon taco seasoning
- 3/4 cup shredded sharp cheddar cheese
- 4 slices of pickled jalapeño
- ¼ cup of salsa
- 3 shredded romaine leaves
- ¼ cup sour cream
- 2/3 cup water

Directions:
1. Grease with oil a skillet of large size, and heat it over medium-high heat.
2. Cook the ground beef in the skillet for 10-15 minutes or until it gives a brownish look.
3. Once the beef gets brown, drain the grease from the skillet and add the water and the taco seasoning.
4. Once the taco seasoning gets mixed well, reduce the heat and simmer for 8-10 minutes.

5. Meanwhile, take both avocados and cut them halves using a sharp knife.
6. Take each avocado shell, fill it with ¼ of the shredded romaine leaves and then fill each shell with ¼ of the cooked ground beef.
7. Topping the avocado taco boats with sour cream, cheese, jalapeno, salsa, and tomato. Serve and Enjoy!

Nutrition: Calories 275, Fat 9,9, Fiber 2,3, Carbs 6,2, Protein 39.

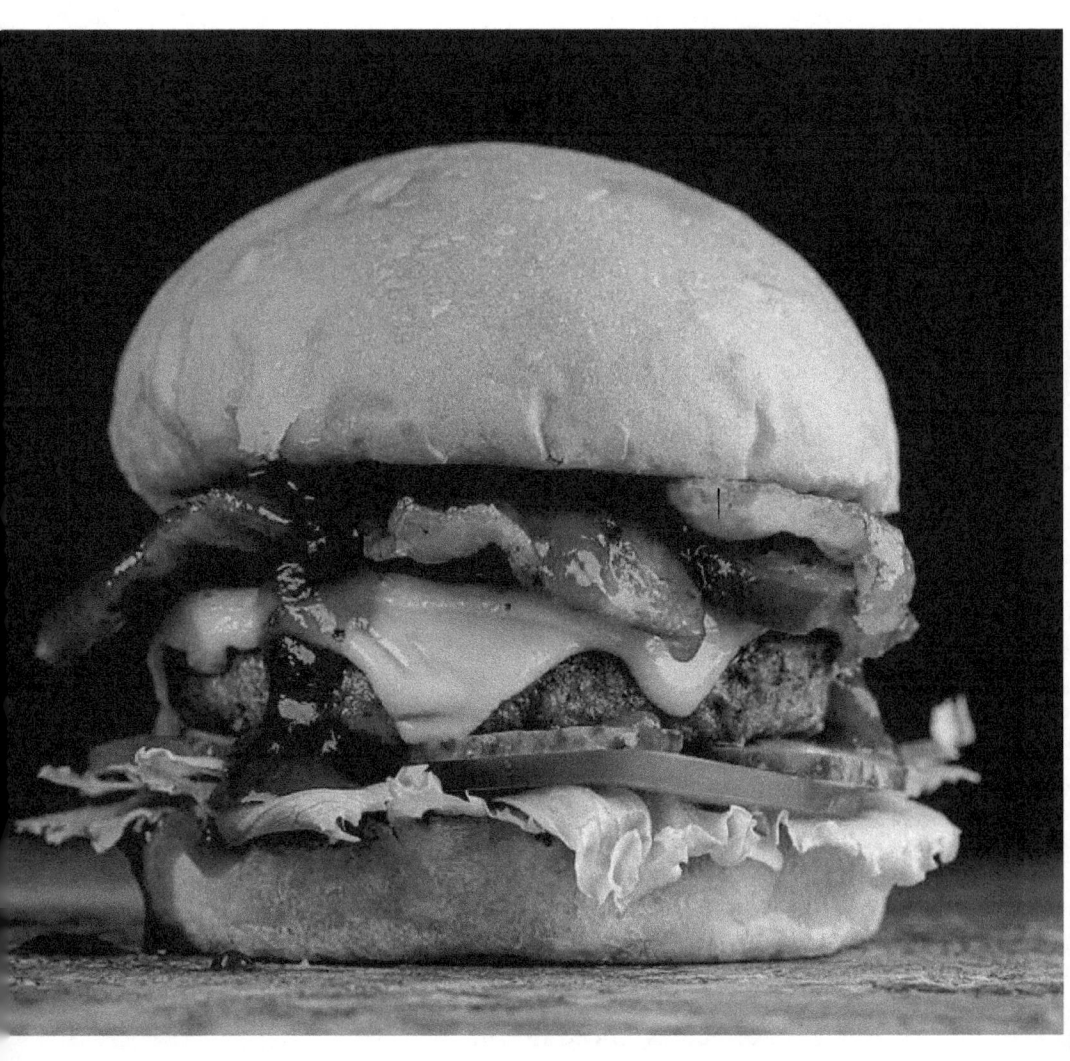

2. Bacon Cheeseburger

Preparation Time: 10 minutes

Cooking Time: 30 minutes

Servings: 4

Ingredients:
- 1 lb. lean ground beef
- ¼ cup chopped yellow onion
- 1 clove garlic, minced
- 1 tbsp. of yellow mustard
- 1 tbsp. of Worcestershire sauce
- ½ tsp. salt
- Cooking spray
- 4 ultra-thin slices of cheddar cheese (cut into 6 equal-sized rectangular pieces)
- 3 pieces of turkey bacon (each cut into 8 evenly-sized rectangular pieces)
- 24 dill pickle chips 4-6 green leaf
- Lettuce leaves
- 12 cherry tomatoes, sliced in half

Directions:

1. Pre-heat oven to 400°F.
2. Into a bowl, combine the garlic, salt, onion, Worcestershire sauce, and beef, mix well, and then form 24 meatballs with your hands.
3. Put meatballs onto a foil-lined baking sheet, bake, and cook for 12-15 minutes.
4. At the end of the time, top every meatball with a piece of cheese and bake again for a few minutes until cheese melts.
5. At this point assemble the skewers inserting one cheese-covered meatball, then a piece of bacon, a piece of lettuce, a pickle chip, and finally a tomato half.
6. You have created a delicious snack! Serve and enjoy!

Nutrition: Calories 252 - Fat 14, Carbs 30, Protein 15.

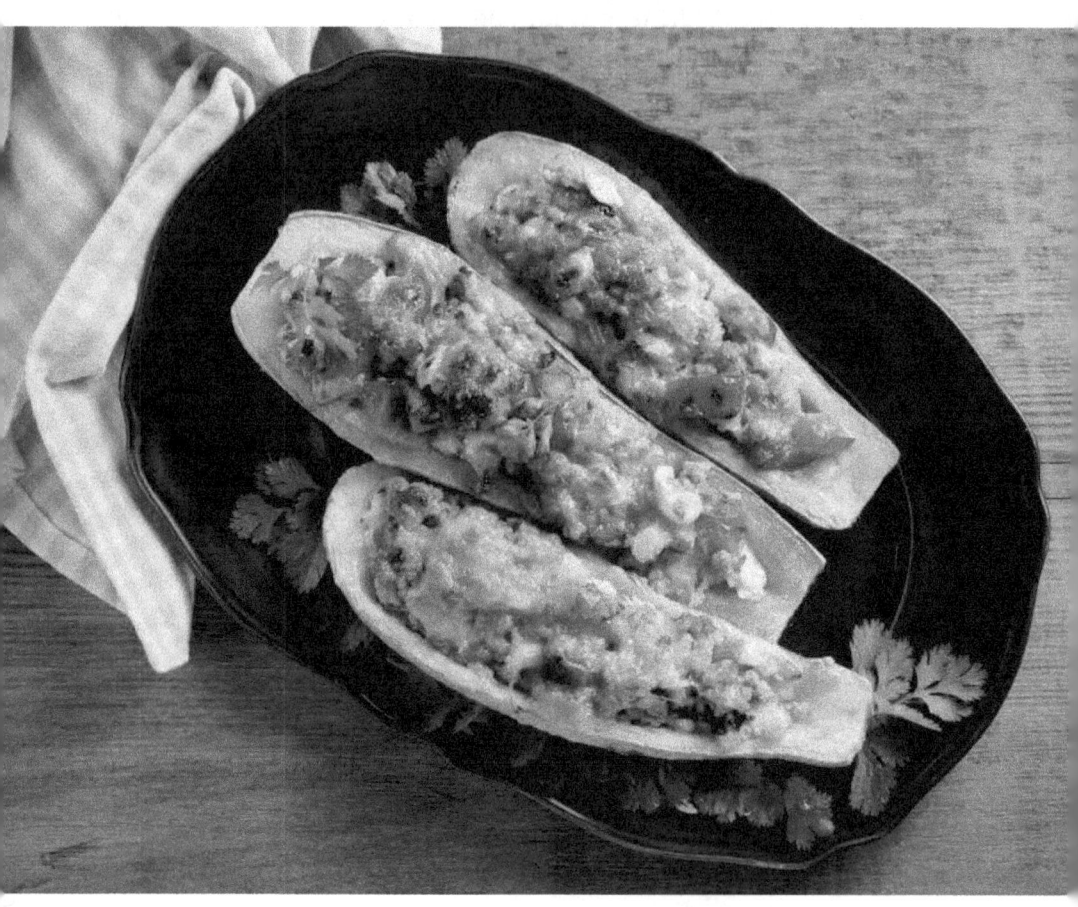

3. Baked Beef Zucchini

Preparation Time: 10 minutes

Cooking Time: 40 minutes

Servings: 4

Ingredients:
- 2 large zucchinis
- 1 cup of minced beef
- 1 cup of mushroom, chopped
- 1 tomato, chopped
- ½ cup of spinach, chopped
- 1 tbsp. of chives, minced
- 2 tbsp. of olive oil
- Salt and pepper to taste
- 1 tbsp. of almond butter
- 1 tsp. of garlic powder
- 1 cup of cheddar cheese, grated
- 1/3 tsp. of ginger powder

Directions:
1. Preheat the oven to 400°F and add aluminum foil on a baking sheet.

2. Cut the zucchini in half, then cut and dig them, putting the filling aside.

3. Add the olive oil in a skillet, heat on medium-high heat, and brown the beef.

4. When the beef is browned, add the mushroom, tomato, chives, salt, pepper, garlic, ginger, and spinach and cook for a few minutes.

5. Stuff the zucchinis using the mixture of meat and vegetables, then add them onto the baking sheet and sprinkle them with the cheese on top.

6. Add a few flakes of butter on top, bake for 30 minutes e finally serve warm. Enjoy!

Nutrition: Cal. 275,1 - Fat 12,7, Carbs 26,8.

4. Cheeseburger Pie

Preparation Time: 20 minutes

Cooking Time: 1 hour 30 minutes

Servings: 4

Ingredients:
- 1 large squash
- 1 lb. lean ground beef
- ¼ cup diced onion
- 2 eggs
- 1/3 cup low-fat, plain Greek yogurt
- 2 tbsp. tomato sauce
- ½ tsp. Worcestershire sauce
- 2/3 cup reduced-fat, shredded cheddar cheese
- 2 oz. dill pickle slices
- Cooking spray

Directions:
1. Preheat the oven to 400°F, line a pan with parchment paper, and grease a pan with cooking spray.
2. Slice squash in half lengthwise, dismiss pulp and seeds, then place the halves cut-side-down in the baking sheet, cover with a foil-lined and bake for 30 minutes.

3. Once the squash is cooked, let cool, and when it's cold, scraping its flesh with a fork and put the squash strands in the greased pan creating an even layer.

4. In a lightly greased, medium-sized skillet, brown beef and onion over medium heat and cook them for about 10 minutes, stirring occasionally.

5. In a bowl, combine eggs, tomato paste, Greek yogurt, and Worcestershire sauce and whisk them. Then, stir in the ground beef mixture.

6. Pour pie filling over squash crust, sprinkle meat filling with cheese, and then top with dill pickle slices.

7. Bake for 40 minutes, then serve and enjoy!

Nutrition: Calories 409, Fat 24,5, Carbs 15, Protein 31.

5. Chocolate Orange Bites

Preparation Time: 20 minutes

Cooking Time: 2 hours

Servings: 6

Ingredients:
- 10 ounces of coconut oil
- 4 tablespoons of cocoa powder
- ¼ teaspoon of orange extract
- Stevia to taste

Directions:
1. Melt half of your coconut oil using a double boiler, and then add in your stevia and orange extract.
2. Pour the mixture into candy molds, filling each mold halfway, and then place in the fridge until they set.
3. After melting the other half of coconut oil, add in the cocoa powder and stevia, and mix until it's smooth.
4. Pour this mix into the molds, filling them up all the way, put in the fridge, and allow it to set before serving.

Nutrition: Calories 188, Fat 21, Carbs 5, Protein 1.

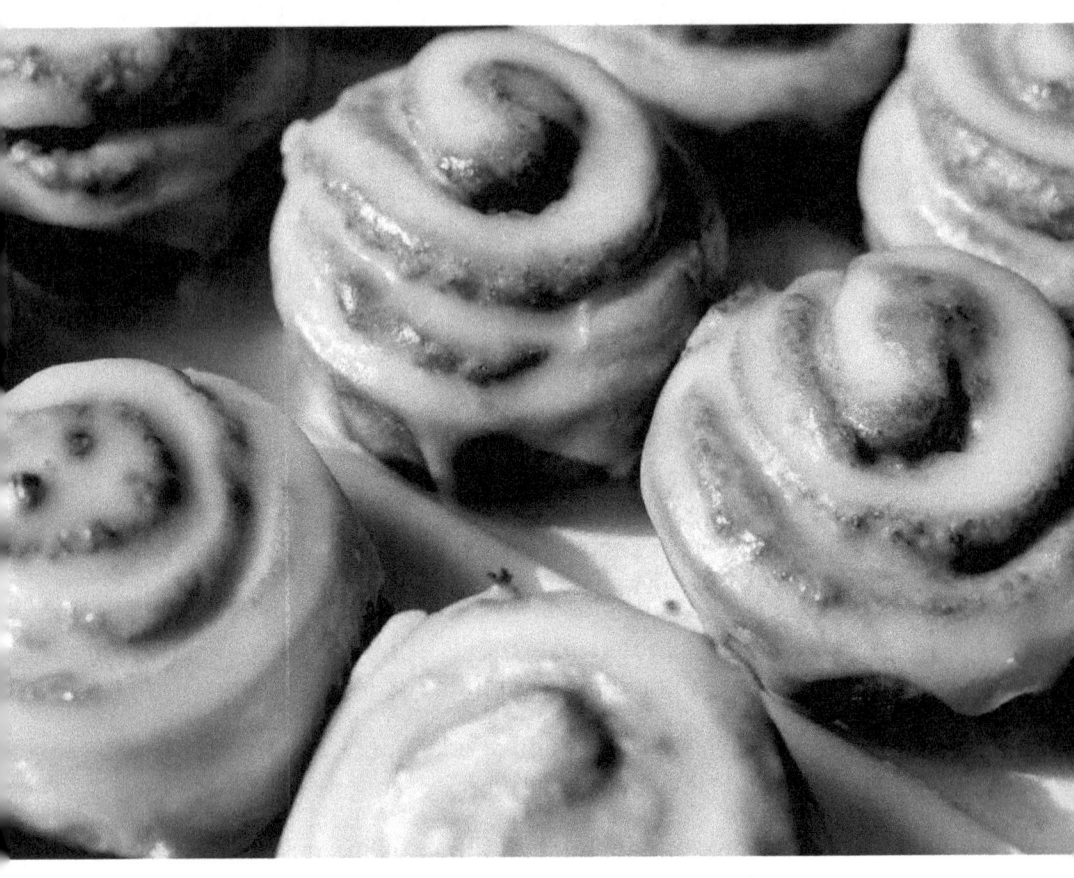

6. Cinnamon Bites

Preparation Time: 20 minutes

Cooking Time: 1 hour 30 minutes

Servings: 6
Ingredients:
- 1/8 teaspoon of nutmeg
- 1 teaspoon of vanilla extract
- ¼ teaspoon of cinnamon
- 4 tablespoons of coconut oil
- ½ cup butter, grass-fed 8 ounces cream cheese Stevia to taste

Directions:
1. Combine the coconut oil, butter, and cream cheese and mix them to soft.
2. Add all of the remaining ingredients, and mix well.
3. Pour the mixture into molds, and freeze until set.

Nutrition: Calories 178, Fat 19, Protein 1.

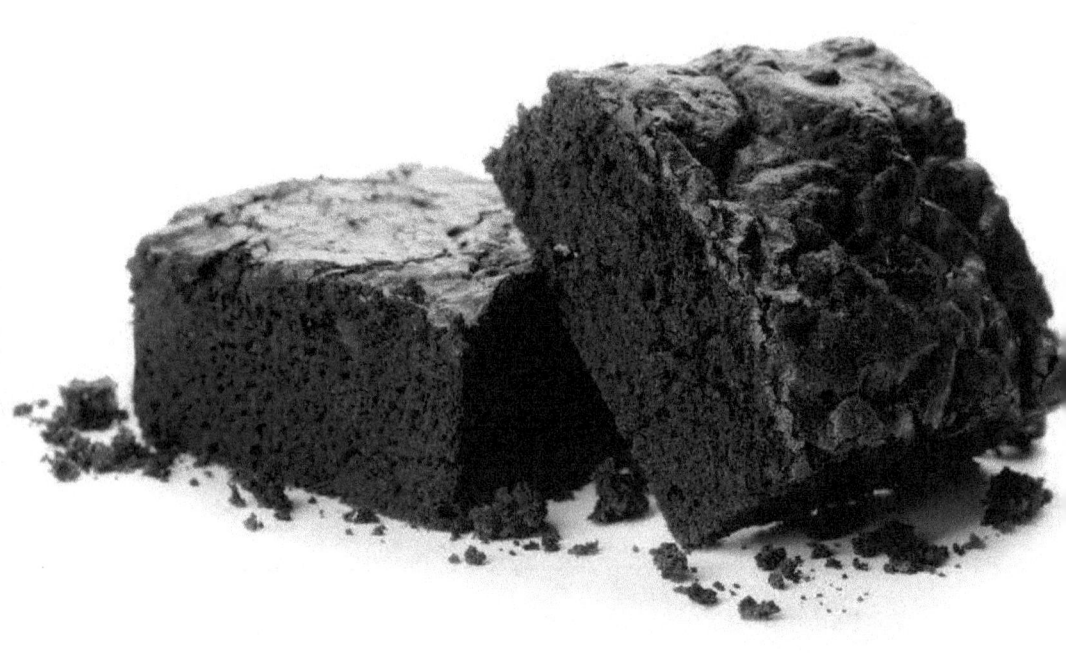

7. Cocoa Brownies

Preparation Time: 10 minutes

Cooking Time: 30 minutes

Servings: 12

Ingredients:
- 1 egg
- 2 tablespoons butter, grass-fed
- 2 teaspoons vanilla extract, pure
- ¼ teaspoon baking powder
- ¼ cup of cocoa powder
- 1/3 cup heavy cream
- ¾ cup almond butter
- Pinch sea salt

Directions:
1. Preheat the oven to 350 degrees and grease a baking pan.
2. Into a bowl, break and whisk an egg, then add in all of your wet ingredients, mixing well.
3. Into another bowl, mix all dry ingredients, then sift them into the first bowl and mix gently without forming a lump.
4. Pour the mixture into the baking pan and bake for about 25 minutes.

5. Remove from the oven, allow it to cool, then slice and serve. Enjoy!

Nutrition: Calories 184, Fat 20, Carbs 1, Protein 1.

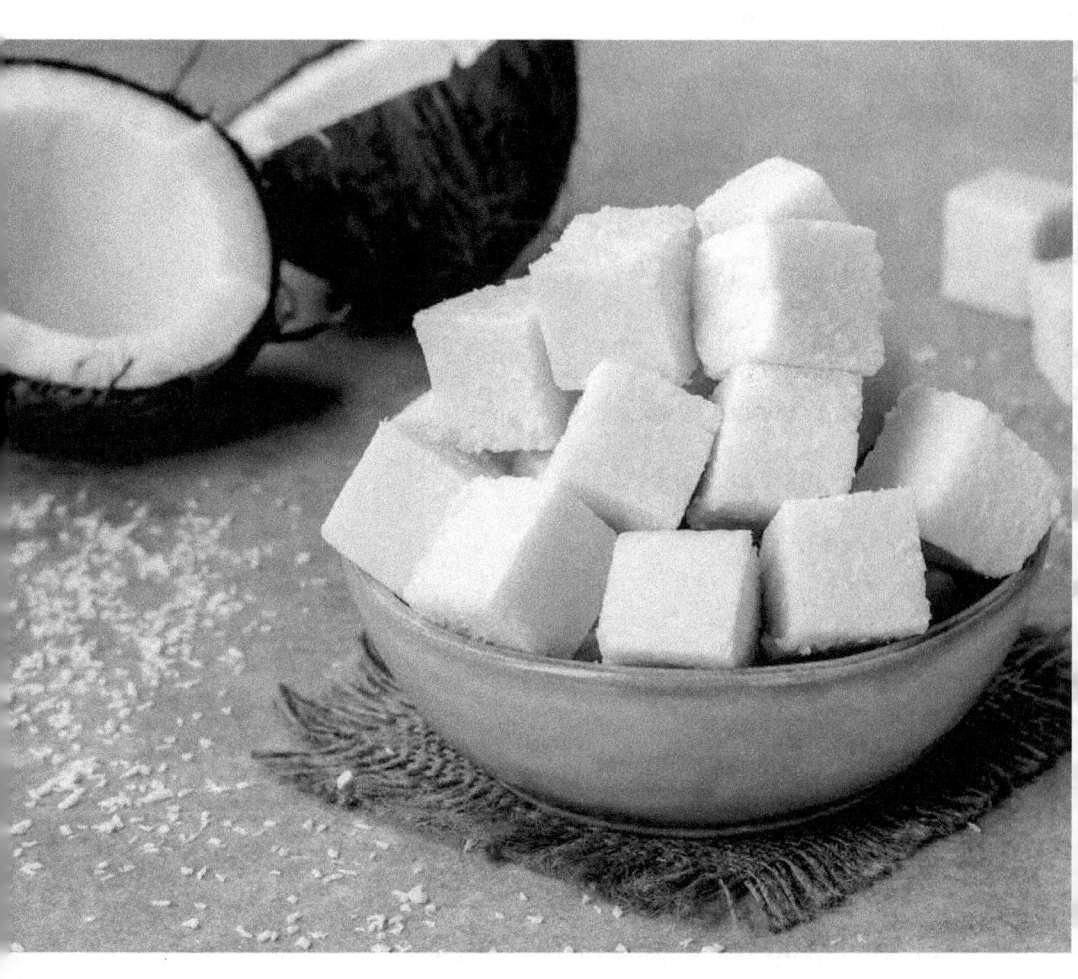

8. Coconut Fudge

Preparation Time: 20 minutes

Cooking Time: 1 hour

Servings: 12

Ingredients:
- 2 cups of coconut oil
- ½ cup dark cocoa powder
- ½ cup coconut cream
- ¼ cup almonds, chopped
- ¼ cup coconut, shredded
- 1 teaspoon almond extract
- Pinch of salt
- Stevia to taste

Directions:
1. Into a bowl, pour your coconut oil and coconut cream and whisk until it's smooth.
2. Add in the cocoa powder mixing slowly, so that no lumps form.
3. Add in the rest of your ingredients, and mix well.
4. Line a pan with parchment paper, pour the mixture on it, and freeze until it sets.
5. Finally, slice into squares and serve.

Nutrition: Calories 172, Fat 20, Protein 3.

9. Easy Vanilla Bombs

Preparation Time: 20 minutes

Cooking Time: 45 minutes

Servings: 14

Ingredients:
- 1 cup of macadamia nuts, unsalted
- ¼ cup of coconut oil / ¼ cup butter
- 2 teaspoons of vanilla extract, sugar-free
- 20 drops liquid Stevia
- 2 tablespoons erythritol, powdered

Directions:
1. In a blender, mince the macadamia nuts, then combine the remaining ingredients and mix well.
2. Using a spoon, put 1 tablespoon and half of the mixture into the cupcake papers.
3. Refrigerate them for a half-hour and finally serve and enjoy!

Nutrition: Calories 125, Fat 5, Carbs 5.

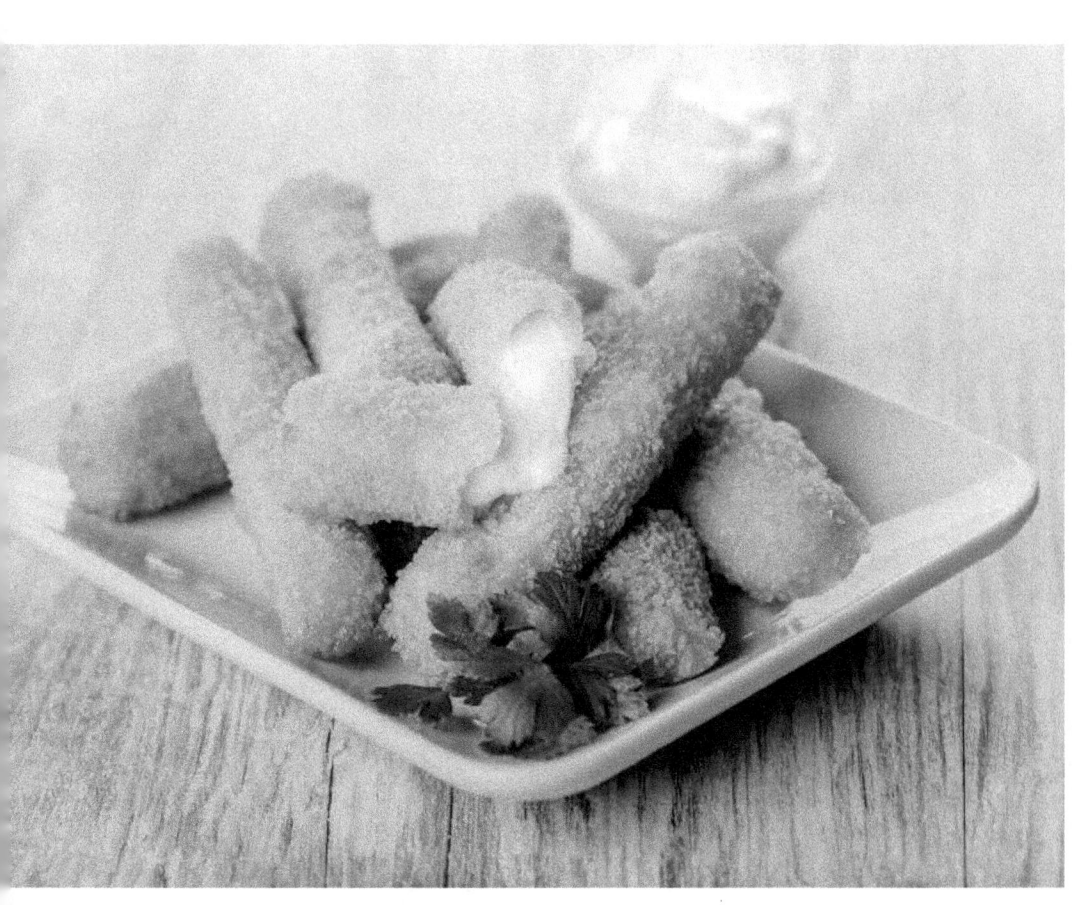

10. Mozzarella Sticks

Preparation Time: 8 minutes

Cooking Time: 2 minutes

Servings: 2

Ingredients:
- 1 large whole egg
- 3 sticks mozzarella cheese in half (frozen overnight)
- 2 tablespoons grated parmesan cheese
- ½ cup of almond flour
- ¼ cup of coconut oil
- 2 ½ teaspoons of Italian seasoning blend
- 1 tablespoon of chopped parsley
- ½ teaspoon of salt

Directions:
1. In a medium skillet, heat the coconut oil over low-medium heat.
2. Into a bowl, crack and whisk the egg.
3. Into another bowl add parmesan cheese, almond flour, and seasonings and whisk them until the mixture is smooth.
4. Dip the overnight frozen mozzarella sticks before in the beaten egg and after in the dry mixture.

5. Place all the coated sticks in the preheated skillet and cook them for 2 minutes or until they start giving a golden-brown look from all sides.

6. When they're cooked, remove them from the skillet and place them over an absorbent paper sheet.

7. If you desire, sprinkle parsley over the sticks and serve with keto marinara sauce. Enjoy!

Nutrition: Calories 430, Fat 39, Carbs 10, Protein 20.

11. Nutmeg Nougat

Preparation Time: 30 minutes

Cooking Time: 1 hour

Servings: 12

Ingredients:
- 1 cup of heavy cream
- 1 cup of cashew butter
- 1 cup of coconut, shredded
- ½ teaspoon of nutmeg
- 1 teaspoon of vanilla extract, pure
- Stevia to taste

Directions:
1. Melt the cashew butter using a double boiler, and then add in your vanilla extract, dairy cream, nutmeg, and stevia and stir well.
2. Remove from heat, allowing it to cool down, and then put it in the fridge for half an hour.
3. Take small portions of the mixture and form them into balls with your hands, then coat them with shredded coconut.
4. Chill in the fridge for at least two hours before serving. Enjoy!

Nutrition: Calories 341, Fat 34, Carbs 5.

12. Personal Pizza Biscuit

Preparation Time: 5 minutes

Cooking Time: 15 minutes

Servings: 1

Ingredients:

    1 sachet select Buttermilk Cheddar Herb Biscuit.

    2 tbsp. of cold water

    2 tbsp. of no-sugar-added tomato sauce

    ¼ cup of reduced-fat shredded cheese

    Cooking spray

Directions:

1. Preheat the oven to 350°F.
2. Mix biscuit and water, spread mixture into a greased, foil-lined circular baking sheet, and bake for 10 minutes.
3. Top with tomato sauce and cheese, and cook for another 5 minutes until cheese is melted.
4. Finally serve hot and enjoy!

Nutrition: Calories 53,1 - Fat 3,5, Protein 3,6.

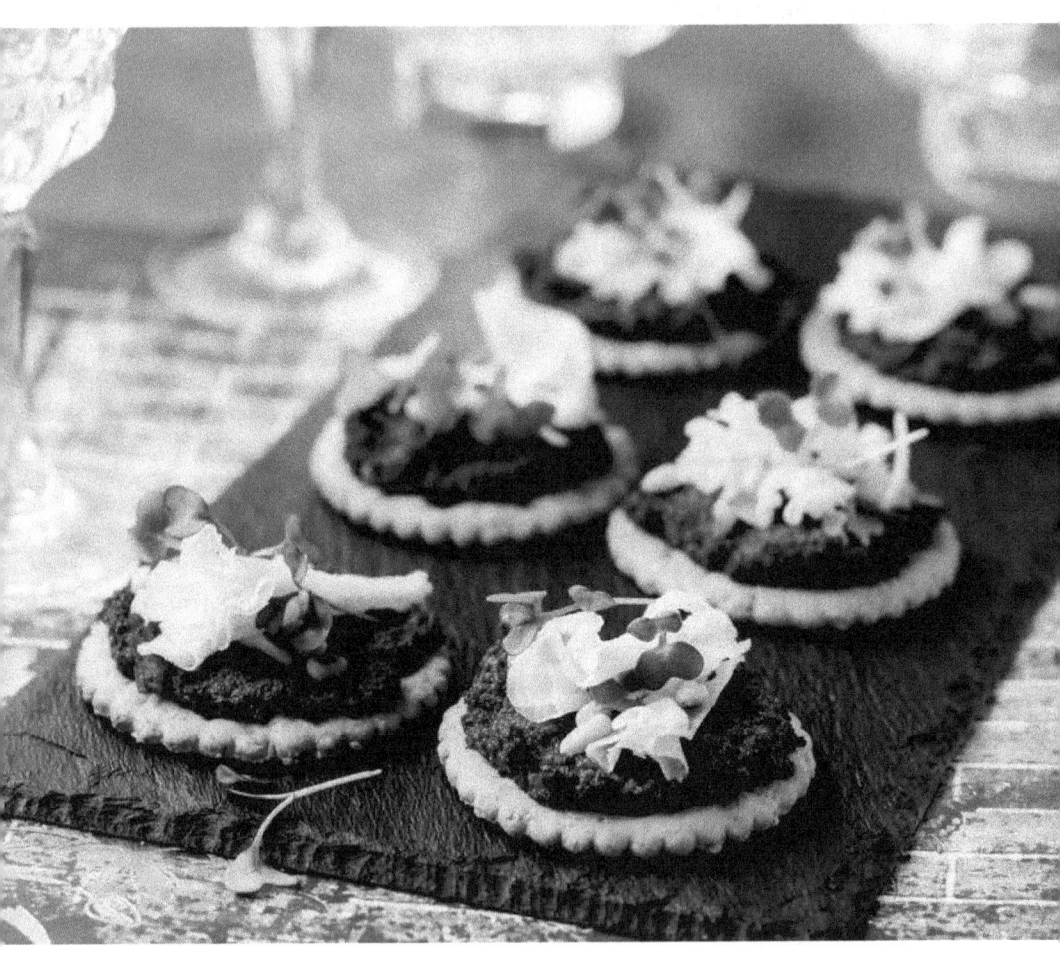

13. Pesto Crackers

Preparation Time: 10 minutes
Cooking Time: 17 minutes
Servings: 6
Ingredients:
- ½ teaspoon baking powder
- 1 ¼ cups almond flour
- ¼ teaspoon basil, dried
- 1 garlic clove, minced
- 2 tablespoons basil pesto
- 3 tablespoons ghee
- A pinch of cayenne pepper
- Salt and black pepper to the taste

Directions:
1. Preheat the oven to 350 degrees.
2. Into a bowl, combine salt, pepper, baking powder, and almond flour and mix.
3. Add in the garlic, cayenne pepper, basil, and stir well, then add in the pesto and whisk.
4. Finally, add in the mixture the ghee and mix the dough with your finger.

5. Spread the dough on a lined baking sheet, introduce in the oven at 325° F and bake for about 17 minutes.

6. After removing it from the oven, leave it aside to cool down.

7. When they're cold, cut the crackers, and serve them as a snack. Enjoy!

Nutrition: Calories 9, Fat 0,1, Carbs 1,8, Protein 0,4.

14. Sausage and Cheese Dip

Preparation Time: 10 minutes

Cooking Time: 2 hours 15 minutes

Servings: 20

Ingredients:
- 8 ounces cream cheese
- 16 ounces sour cream
- 8 ounces pepper jack cheese, chopped
- 15 ounces canned tomatoes mixed with habaneros
- 1-pound Italian sausage, ground
- ¼ cup green onions, chopped
- A pinch of salt and black pepper

Directions:
1. Heat a skillet over medium heat, add sausage, and cook until it browns, stirring occasionally.
2. When it's brown, add in the tomatoes mix, stir and cook for another 4 minutes.
3. Season with a pinch of salt, pepper, add the green onions, stir and cook for 4 minutes more.
4. Meanwhile, on the bottom of a slow cooker, spread the pepper jack cheese, then add in the cream cheese, sausage mix, and sour cream, cover and cook on high heat for about 2 hours.

5. At the end of cooking, stir, transfer to a bowl, and serve. Enjoy!

Nutrition: Calories 132, Fat 9,6, Carbs 6,3, Protein 6,8.

15. Steak and Avocado Lettuce Wraps

Preparation Time: 20 minutes

Cooking Time: 15 minutes

Servings: 8

Ingredients:
- 1 lb. trifecta steak, diced
- 1 large head of Boston lettuce, washed, pat dried, and leaves separated
- 2 medium avocado
- ½ cup of favorite salsa, Store Bought
- ½ teaspoon of kosher salt
- ½ tsp. black pepper
- 1 tbsp. of coriander seed
- ½ tsp. of garlic powder
- 1 tbsp. of coconut oil
- favorite toppings of choice

Directions:
1. Wash, dry and separate the leaves of 1 large lettuce head of large leaf and set aside.

2. In a skillet, heat coconut oil over medium low heat, add the spices in and slightly 'toast' them until aromatic.

3. Increase the heat to medium high, add the diced protein and sauté for 3-5 minutes, until protein is warm.

4. In a small bowl, crush the pulp of two avocados with a fork until just creamy and then season with salt, and lime juice.

5. Into each piece of lettuce spread avocado cream with equally protein and top with your favorite salsa to taste.

6. Finally, fold like a taco and enjoy!

Note: You can use any favorite toppings like chopped tomatoes, diced onions, and cilantro.

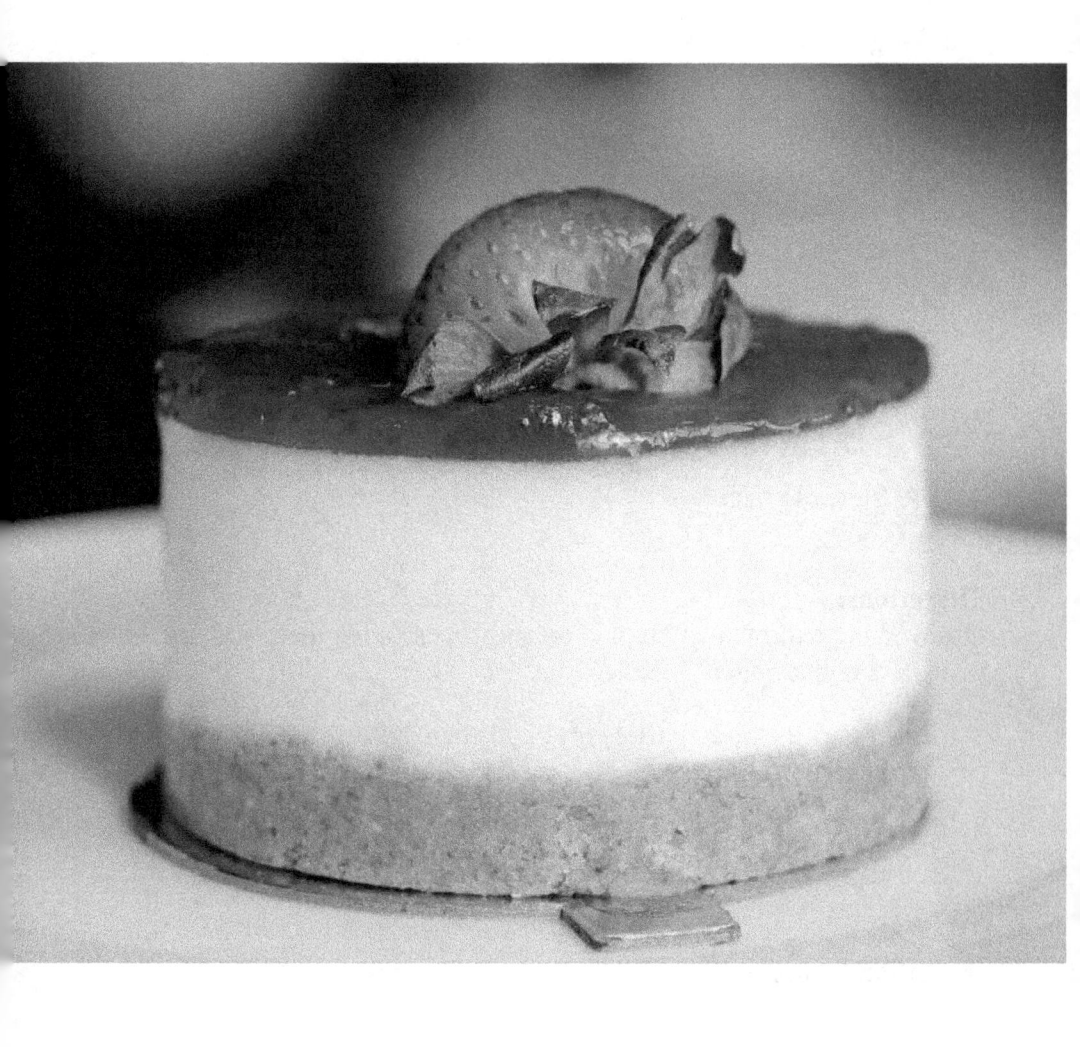

16. Strawberry Cheesecake Minis

Preparation Time: 30 minutes

Cooking Time: 2 hours

Servings: 12

Ingredients:
- 1 cup of coconut oil
- 1 cup of coconut butter
- ½ cup strawberries, sliced
- ½ teaspoon lime juice
- 2 tablespoons of cream cheese
- Stevia to taste

Directions:
1. Into a bowl soften the cream cheese and then add in the coconut butter.
2. Blend the strawberries and add them into the bowl with the cheese cream.
3. Mix it, pour the mixture into silicone molds and freeze for at least two hours before serving.

Nutrition: Calories 372, Fat 41, Carbs 2, Protein 1.

17. Sweet Almond Bites

Preparation Time: 30 minutes

Cooking Time: 1 hour 30 minutes

Servings: 12
Ingredients:
- 18 ounces butter, grass-fed
- 2 ounces heavy cream
- ½ cup Stevia
- 2/3 cup cocoa powder
- 1 teaspoon vanilla extract, pure
- 4 tablespoons almond butter

Directions:
1. Melt the butter in a double boiler and then add in all of the remaining ingredients.
2. Place the mixture into molds and leave to rest in the freezer for two hours before serving.

Nutrition: Calories 350, Fat 38, Protein 2.

18. Sweet Chai Bites

Preparation Time: 20 minutes

Cooking Time: 45 minutes

Servings: 6

Ingredients:
- 1 cup of cream cheese
- 1 cup of coconut oil
- 2 ounces butter, grass-fed
- 2 teaspoons ginger
- 2 teaspoons cardamom
- 1 teaspoon nutmeg
- 1 teaspoon cloves
- 1 teaspoon vanilla extract, pure
- 1 teaspoon Darjeeling black tea
- Stevia to taste

Directions:
1. Melt the coconut oil and butter in a double boiler, and then add in the black tea and let it rest for one to two minutes.
2. Remove the mixture from the heat and add in the cream cheese stirring gently.
3. Finally, add in all spices, and stir to combine.

4. Pour into molds, and freeze them for two hours before serving.

Nutrition: Calories 178, Fat 19, Protein 1.

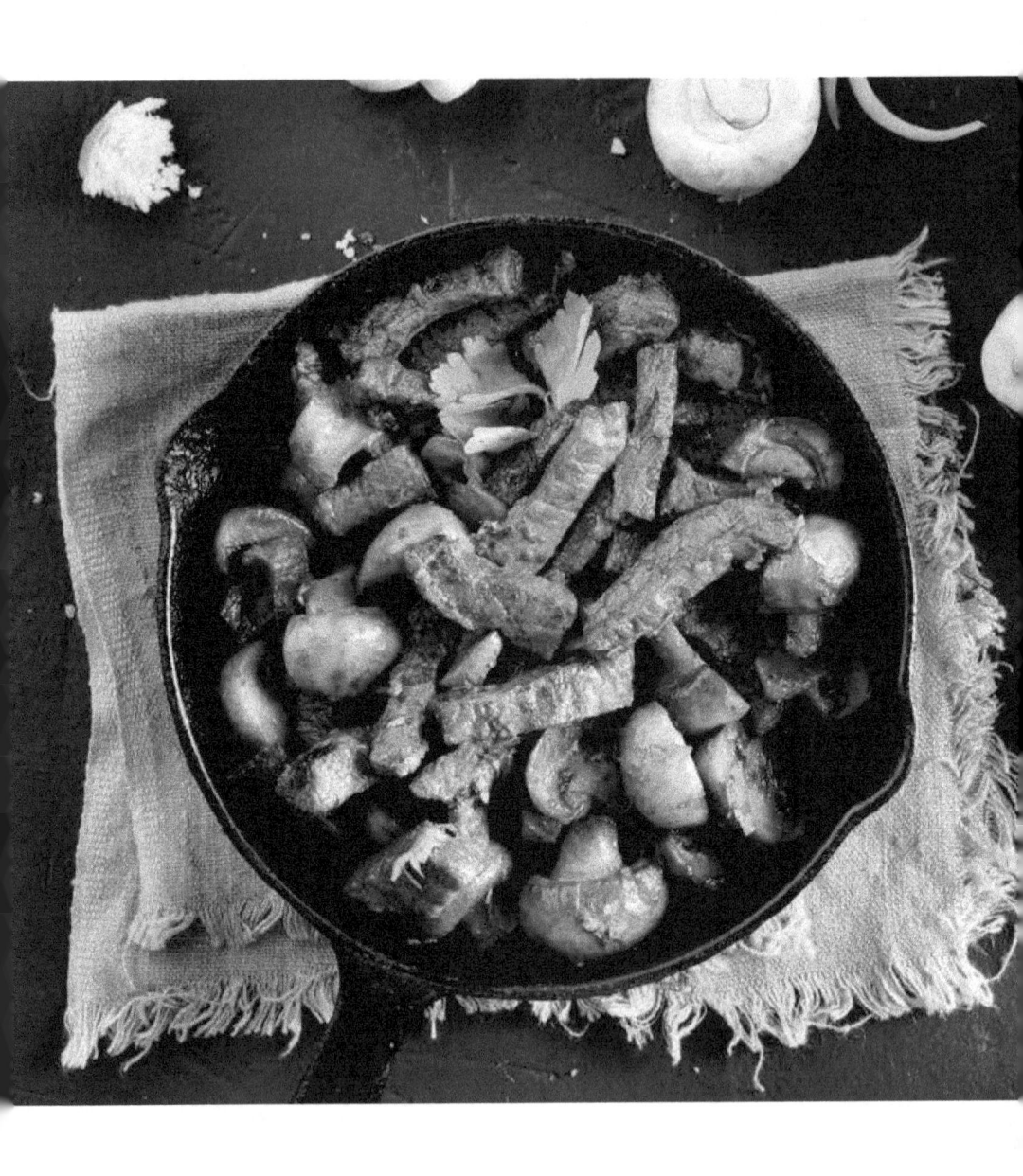

19. Beef and Mushrooms

Preparation time: 10 minutes

Cooking time: 25 minutes

Servings: 4

Ingredients:
- 1 ½ lb lean beef (chop into 1-inch chunks)
- ½ tablespoon of garlic seasoning (or mixture of garlic, salt, and pepper)
- 4 cups of mushrooms
- 1 cup of beef broth (low sodium)
- 1 ½ teaspoon of garlic and spring onion seasoning (or a mixture of parsley, fresh garlic, and onion)

Directions:
1. Into a bowl, add the beef and seasoning and toss to coat completely.
2. Grease a pan with nonstick cooking spray and heat on over high heat.
3. In a single layer, add the seasoned beef to the pan and brown for about 7 minutes for each side or until it turns brown.
4. Remove the pork from heat and transfer it onto a bowl, covering with a kitchen towel and keeping it warm.
5. Reduce the heat to medium-high and add the broth to the pan.
6. Scrape the brown bits from the bottom of the pan with your wooden spoon, add the garlic seasoning and mushrooms and simmer until the mixture reduces by half.

7. Return the beef into the pan and toss to combine well, then serve.

Nutrition: Calories 254, Fat 10,8, Fiber 0,7, Carbs 2,3, Protein 35,5.

20. Beef Stroganoff

Preparation Time: 10 minutes

Cooking Time: 8 hours

Servings: 2

Ingredients:
- ½ lb. beef stew meat
- 10 oz. mushroom soup, homemade
- 1 medium onion, chopped
- ½ cup sour cream
- 2.5 oz. mushrooms, sliced
- Pepper and salt

Directions:
1. Add all ingredients except sour cream into the crockpot and mix well.
2. Cover and cook slowly on low heat for 8 hours.
3. When the stew is cooked, add sour cream, stir well and serve. Enjoy!

Nutrition: Calories 470, Fat 25, Carbs 8,6, Protein 49.

21. Cayenne Rib Eye Steak

Preparation Time: 10 minutes

Cooking Time: 13 minutes

Servings: 2

Ingredients:
- 1-pound rib-eye steak
- 1 teaspoon of salt
- 1 teaspoon of cayenne pepper
- ½ teaspoon chili flakes
- 3 tablespoon cream
- 1 teaspoon olive oil
- 1 teaspoon lemongrass
- 1 tablespoon butter
- 1 teaspoon garlic powder

Directions:
1. Preheat the air fryer to 360 °F.
2. Into a small bowl, combine the cayenne pepper, salt, chili flakes, lemongrass, and garlic powder, mix gently and sprinkle the rib eye steak with the spice mixture.
3. Melt the butter and combine it with cream and olive oil.
4. Churn the mixture and pour it into the air fryer basket tray.

5. Add the rib eye steak and cook it for 13 minutes without turning it.

6. When the steak is cooked, transfer it to a paper towel to soak all the excess fat, then slice it and serve! Enjoy!

Nutrition: Calories 708, Fat 59, Carbs 2,3, Protein 40,4.

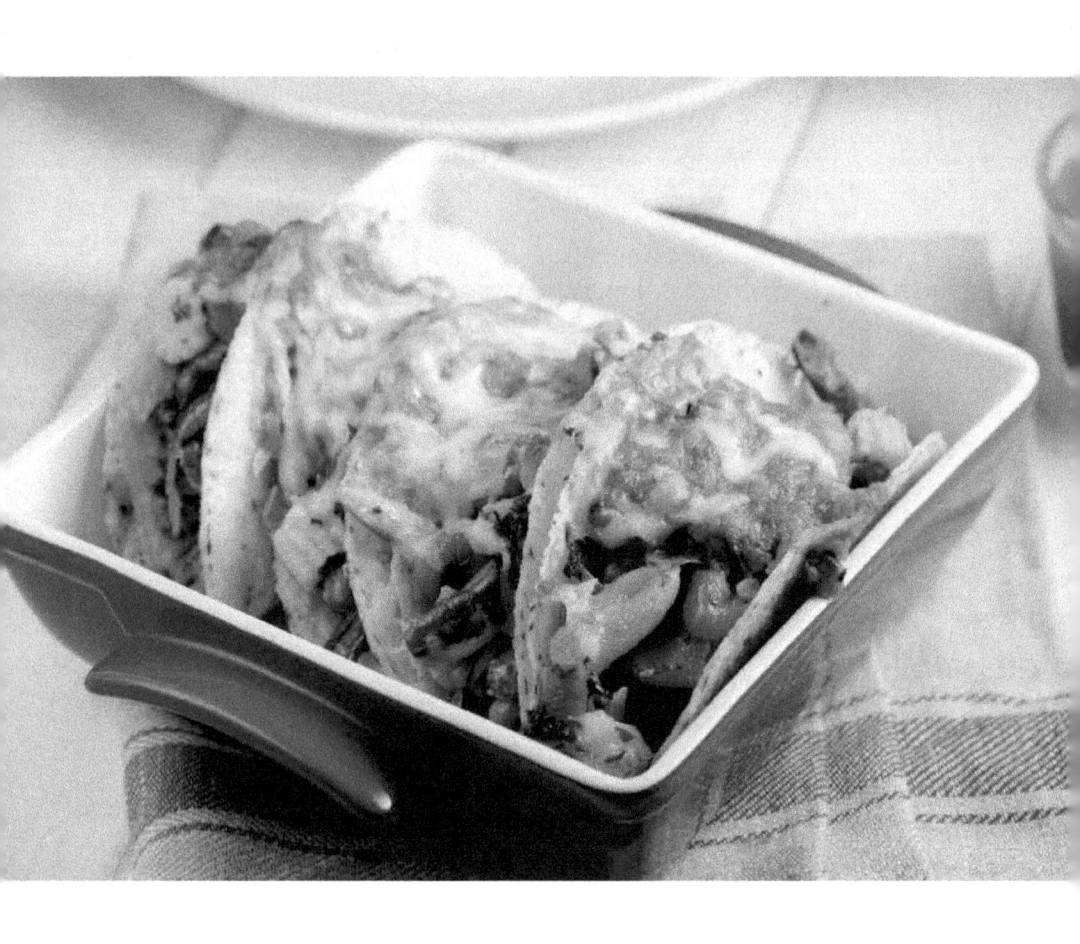

22. Cheesy Taco Bake

Preparation Time: 10 minutes

Cooking Time: 30 minutes

Servings: 4

Ingredients:
- 1 lb 96-98% lean ground beef (turkey or chicken) - 1lb
- 1 tablespoon of seasoning mix (with garlic, paprika, cayenne, cumin, salt, onion, black pepper, and/or parsley)
- 1 cup of fresh vegetable salsa (with no sugar added) plus extra 4 tablespoons for garnish
- 1 ½ lb of fresh peppers (cut lengthwise and seeded -
- ½ cup of low-fat cheddar cheese (shredded)
- 4 tablespoons of sour cream

Directions:
1. Preheat the oven to 350 degrees.
2. Into a bowl, add the salsa, meat, and seasonings and mix thoroughly with your fingers.
3. Then, equally divide the mixture and stuff the pepper halves.
4. Place the stuffed peppers in a baking dish, sprinkle over with cheese and bake in the oven for about 30 min.
5. Remove from the oven and make 4 serves with 1 tablespoon of salsa and sour cream on the top of each one. Enjoy!

Nutrition: Calories 319, Fat 12,2, Fiber 2,6, Carbs 9,1, Protein 42,6.

23. Chili Beef Jerky

Preparation Time: 25 minutes

Cooking Time: 2 hours 30 minutes

Servings: 6

Ingredients:
- 14 oz. beef flank steak
- 1 teaspoon chili pepper
- 3 tablespoon apple cider vinegar
- 1 teaspoon ground black pepper
- 1 teaspoon onion powder
- 1 teaspoon garlic powder
- ¼ teaspoon liquid smoke

Directions:
1. Into a bowl combine the apple cider vinegar, ground black pepper, onion powder, garlic powder, and liquid smoke and whisk gently with a fork.
2. Slice the beefsteak into medium strips, tenderize each piece and dip them in the mixture, stirring well.
3. Leave the meat to marinate for up to eight hours in the fridge.
4. Preheat the air fryer to 150° and then put the marinated beef pieces in the air fryer rack.

5. Cook the beef jerky for 2 hours and 30 minutes at 150 °F and finally serve!

Nutrition: Calories 129, Fat 4,1, Carbs 1,1, Protein 20,2.

24. Greek Beef Roast

Preparation Time: 10 minutes

Cooking Time: 8 hours

Servings: 6

Ingredients:
- 2 lbs. lean top round beef roast
- 1 tablespoon Italian seasoning
- 6 garlic cloves, minced
- 1 onion, sliced
- 2 cups of beef broth
- ½ cup of red wine
- 1 teaspoon of red pepper flakes
- Pepper and salt

Directions:
1. Season meat with pepper and salt and place into the crockpot.
2. Pour remaining ingredients over meat, cover, and cook slowly on low heat for 8 hours.
3. When the stew is ready, shred the meat using a fork, serve, and enjoy.

Nutrition: Calories 231, Fat 6, Carbs 4, Protein 35.

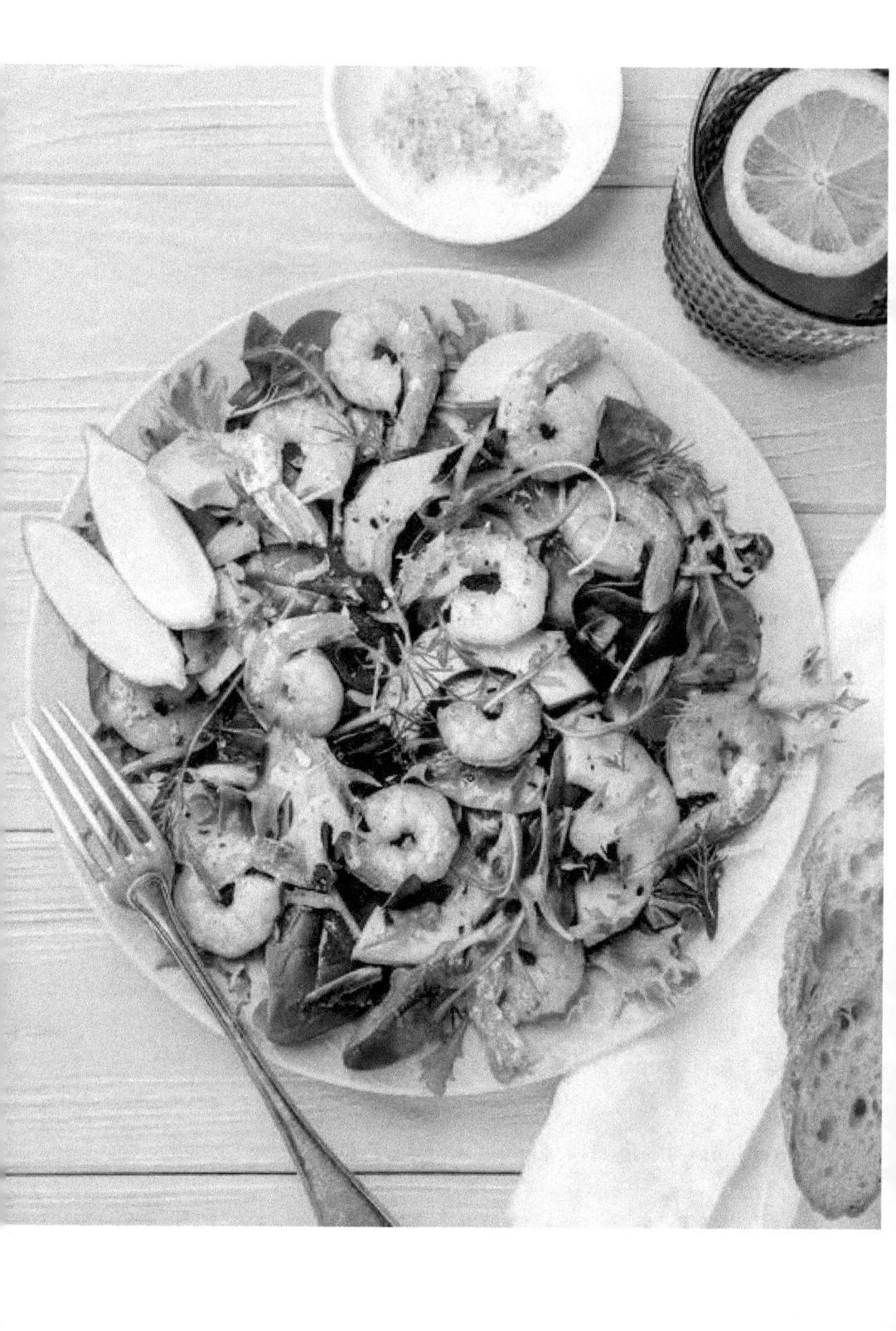

25. Avocado Lime Shrimp Salad

Preparation time: 15 minutes

Cooking time: 0 minutes

Servings: 2
Ingredients:
- 14 ounces of jumbo cooked shrimp, peeled and deveined; chopped
- 4 ½ ounces of avocado, diced
- 1 ½ cup of tomato, diced
- ¼ cup of chopped green onion
- ¼ cup of jalapeno with the seeds removed, finely diced
- 1 teaspoon of olive oil
- 2 tablespoons of lime juice
- 1/8 teaspoon of salt
- 1 tablespoon of chopped cilantro

Directions:
1. In a small bowl combine green onion, olive oil, lime juice, pepper, and a pinch of salt and marinate the ingredients for about 5 minutes.
2. In a large bowl combine chopped shrimp, tomato, avocado, jalapeno, and cilantro, and gently toss.
3. Add pepper and salt as desired and serve.

Nutrition: Calories 314, Fat 9, Carbs 15, Protein 2.

26. Baked Cod Crusted with Herbs

Preparation Time: 5 minutes

Cooking Time: 10 minutes

Servings: 4

Ingredients:
- ¼ cup honey
- ¼ teaspoon salt
- ½ cup panko
- ½ teaspoon pepper
- 1 tablespoon extra-virgin olive oil
- 1 tablespoon lemon juice
- 1 teaspoon dried basil
- 1 teaspoon dried parsley
- 1 teaspoon rosemary
- 4 pieces of 4-oz cod fillets

Directions:
1. Preheat the oven to 375°F and grease a 9 x 13-inch baking pan with olive oil.
2. In a zip-lock bag, mix panko, rosemary, salt, pepper, parsley, and basil.

3. Evenly spread cod fillets in a dish, drizzle with lemon juice, and then brush the fillets with honey on all sides.

4. Divide the panko mixture on top of cod fillets and bake for 10 minutes or until fish is cooked.

5. Remove from the oven, serve, and enjoy.

Nutrition: Calories 137, Fat 2, Carbs 21, Protein 5.

27. Baked Tuna with Asparagus

Preparation Time: 10 minutes

Cooking Time: 10 minutes

Servings: 2

Ingredients:
- 2 tuna steak
- 1 cup of asparagus, trimmed
- 1 tsp. almond butter
- 1 tsp. rosemary
- ½ tsp. of oregano
- ½ tsp. garlic powder
- 1 tsp. lemon juice
- ½ tsp. ginger powder
- 1 tbsp. of olive oil
- 1 tsp. of red chili powder
- Salt and pepper to taste

Directions:
1. Marinate the tuna using oregano, lemon juice, salt, pepper, red chili powder, garlic, ginger, and let it sit for 10 minutes.

2. Meanwhile, in a pan melt the almond butter, add the asparagus, salt, pepper, and rosemary and cook for about 10-15 minutes (If necessary, add a little water).

3. Heat another skillet with the olive oil and fry the tuna steaks for 2 minutes per side.

4. Finally serve the tuna steaks with asparagus as a side dish. Enjoy!

Nutrition: Calories 61,5 - Fat 4,7, Carbs 3,2.

28. Cajun Garlic Shrimp Noodle Bowl

Preparation Time: 10 minutes

Cooking Time: 15 minutes

Servings: 2

Ingredients:
- ½ teaspoon salt
- 1 onion, sliced
- 1 red pepper, sliced
- 1 tablespoon butter
- 1 teaspoon garlic granules
- 1 teaspoon onion powder
- 1 teaspoon paprika
- 2 large zucchinis, cut into noodle strips
- 20 jumbo shrimps, shells removed and deveined
- 3 cloves garlic, minced
- 3 tablespoon ghee
- A dash of cayenne pepper
- A dash of red pepper flakes

Directions:

1. Prepare the Cajun seasoning by mixing the onion powder, garlic granules, pepper flakes, cayenne pepper, paprika, and salt.
2. Toss in the shrimp and coat them in the seasoning.
3. In a skillet, heat the ghee and sauté the garlic, then, add in the red pepper and onions and continue sautéing for 4 minutes.
4. Add the Cajun shrimp to the skillet and cook them until opaque. Then, set aside.
5. In another pan, heat the butter and sauté the zucchini noodles for 3 minutes.
6. Serve the zucchini noodles with the Cajun shrimps on top.

Nutrition: Calories 712, Fat 30, Carbs 20,2, Protein 97,8.

29. Caribbean Steamed Fish

Preparation Time: 5 minutes

Cooking Time: 20 minutes

Servings: 8-10

Ingredients:
- 2 lbs fish (porgy or snapper), cleaned and scaled
- Juice of 1 lime
- ½ tsp black pepper
- 1 tsp salt
- 3 cloves garlic – 2 sliced and 1 crushed
- About 15 sprigs thyme
- ½ tbsp butter
- ½ tbsp oil
- 2 carrots, thinly sliced
- 1 red pepper, thinly sliced
- 1 green pepper, thinly sliced
- 1 onion, thinly sliced
- 12 okra, ends cut off
- 1 hot pepper (scotch bonnet, habanero or wiri wiri), seeds removed
- 1 ½ cup water

Directions:
1. Season the fish with lime juice, crushed garlic, black pepper, salt and half of the thyme and set aside.

2. In a large pot, add oil and butter and heat over medium heat. Then, sauté the carrots, red and green pepper, and onion for about 5 minutes, until it has softened.

3. Add garlic slices and pepper and cook for just a 2 minutes.

4. Add water, bring it to boil, and then add fish, okra, and the rest of the thyme into the pot.

5. Lower the heat and cook for 15 minutes until the fish is done, then serve hot.

Nutrition: Calories 378, Fat 7,4, Fiber 3,3, Carbs 13,1, Protein 60,5.

30. Coconut Salsa on Chipotle Fish Tacos

Preparation Time: 10 minutes

Cooking Time: 10 minutes

Servings: 4

Ingredients:
- ¼ cup chopped fresh cilantro
- ½ cup seeded and finely chopped plum tomato
- 1 cup peeled and finely chopped mango
- 1 lime cut into wedges
- 1 tablespoon chipotle Chile powder
- 1 tablespoon safflower oil
- 1/3 cup finely chopped red onion
- 10 tablespoon fresh lime juice, divided
- 4 6-oz boneless, skinless cod fillets
- 5 tablespoon dried unsweetened shredded coconut
- 8 pcs of 6-inch tortillas, heated

Directions:
1. In a glass baking dish, whisk well Chile powder, oil, and four tablespoon lime juice.
2. Add cod and marinate for 12–15 minutes, turning once halfway through the marinating time.

3. In a medium bowl, mixing coconut, 6 tablespoon lime juice, cilantro, onions, tomatoes, and mangoes and set aside.

4. Heat a grill pan on high, place cod, and grill for four minutes per side.

5. Once it's cooked, slice cod into large flakes and evenly divide onto the tortilla.

6. Serve the tortilla with the salsa on top of cod and with lime wedges on the side.

Nutrition: Calories 477, Fat 12,4, Carbs 57,4, Protein 35.

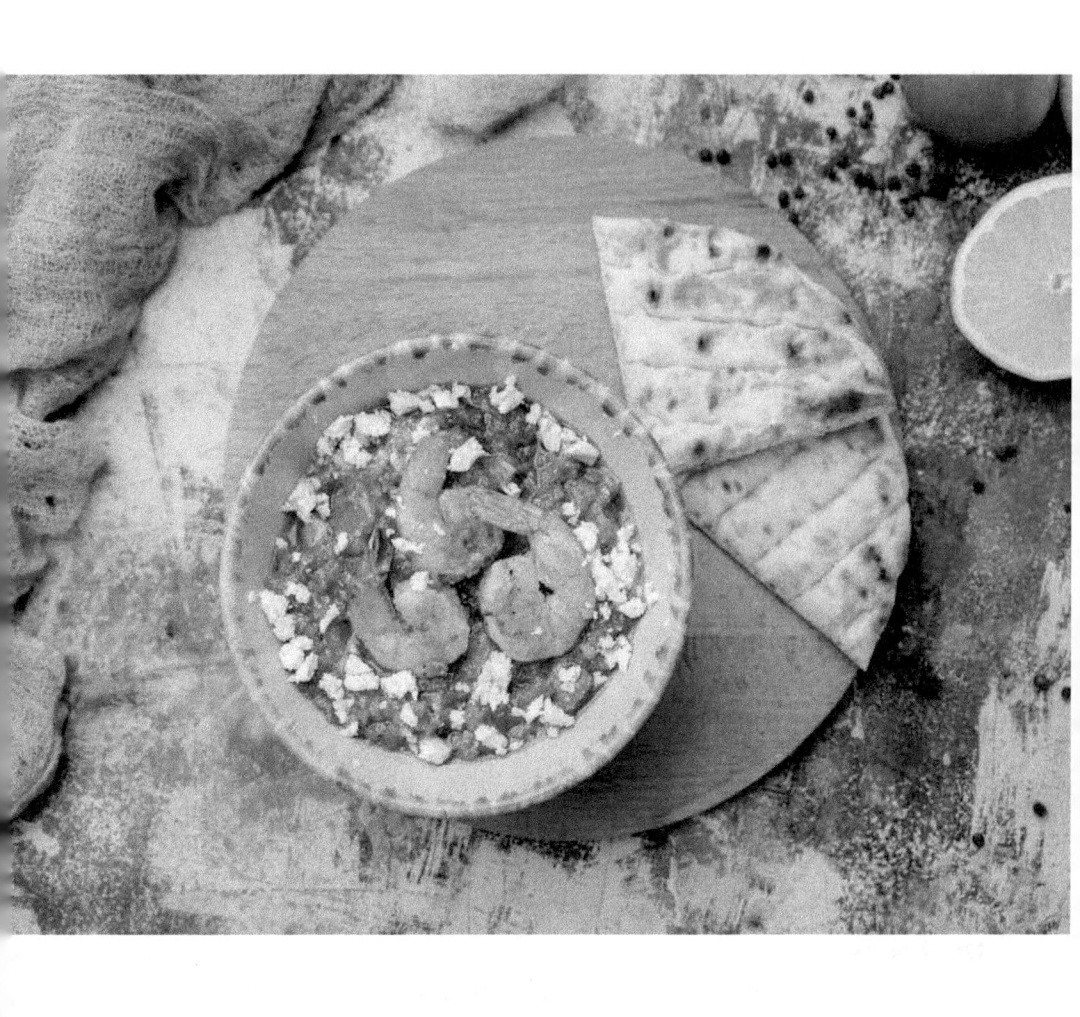

31. Crazy Saganaki Shrimp

Preparation Time: 10 minutes

Cooking Time: 10 minutes

Servings: 4

Ingredients:
- ¼ teaspoon salt
- ½ cup Chardonnay
- ½ cup crumbled Greek feta cheese
- 1 medium bulb. fennel, cored and finely chopped
- 1 small Chile pepper, seeded and minced
- 1 tablespoon extra-virgin olive oil
- 12 jumbo shrimps, deveined with tails left on
- 2 tablespoon lemon juice, divided
- 5 scallions sliced thinly
- Pepper to taste

Directions:
1. In a medium bowl, mix salt, lemon juice, and shrimp.
2. Place a saganaki pan (or large nonstick saucepan) and heat oil on medium heat.
3. Sauté Chile pepper, scallions, and fennel for about 4 minutes.
4. Add wine and let it evaporate for another minute.

5. Place shrimps on top of the fennel, cover, and cook for 4 minutes or until shrimps are pink, then remove just the shrimp and transfer to a plate.

6. Add pepper, feta, and 1 tablespoon lemon juice to the pan and cook for a minute or until the cheese begins to melt.

7. Place the cheese and fennel mixture on a serving plate and top with shrimps.

Nutrition: Calories 310, Fat 6,8, Carbs 8,4, Protein 49,7.

32. Creamy Bacon-Fish Chowder

Preparation Time: 10 minutes

Cooking Time: 30 minutes

Servings: 8

Ingredients:
- 1 ½ lb. cod
- 1 ½ teaspoon dried thyme
- 1 large onion, chopped
- 1 medium carrot, coarsely chopped
- 1 tablespoon butter, cut into small pieces
- 1 teaspoon salt, divided
- 3 ½ cups baking potato, peeled and cubed
- 3 slices uncooked bacon
- 3/4 teaspoon ground black pepper, divided
- 4 ½ cups water
- 4 bay leaves
- 4 cups 2% reduced-fat milk

Directions:
1. In a large skillet, add the water and bay leaves and let it simmer.

2. When it boils, add the fish, cover it, and let it simmer until it becomes soft.

3. Remove the fish from the skillet, cut it into large pieces, and set the cooking liquid aside.

4. In a skillet, cook the bacon on medium heat until crisp. Then remove the bacon, dripping it, and finally crush it and set aside.

5. In the pan stir the potato, onion, and carrots and cook them over medium heat for 10 minutes.

6. Add the cooking liquid, bay leaves, ½ teaspoon salt, ¼ teaspoon pepper, and thyme, let it boil. Then, lower the heat and let simmer for 11 minutes.

7. Add the milk and butter and simmer until the potatoes become tender, then add the fish, ½ teaspoon salt, ½ teaspoon pepper.

8. Remove the bay leaves and serve the fish sprinkled with the crushed bacon.

Nutrition: Calories 400, Fat 19,7, Carbs 34,5, Protein 20,8.

33. Crisped Coco-Shrimp with Mango Dip

Preparation Time: 10 minutes

Cooking Time: 20 minutes

Servings: 4

Ingredients:
- 1 cup of shredded coconut
- 1 lb. raw shrimp, peeled and deveined
- 2 egg whites
- 4 tablespoons of tapioca starch
- Pepper and salt to taste

MANGO DIP INGREDIENTS:
- 1 cup of mango, chopped
- 1 jalapeño, thinly minced
- 1 teaspoon of lime juice
- 1/3 cup coconut milk
- 3 teaspoons of raw honey

Directions:
1. Preheat the oven to 400°F and arrange a pan with a wire rack on top.
2. In a medium bowl, add tapioca starch and season with pepper and salt.
3. In another medium bowl, add egg whites and whisk.

4. In a third medium bowl, add coconut.

5. Dip shrimps first in tapioca starch, then in egg whites, and then in coconut.

6. Place breaded shrimp on the wire rack and roast them for 10 minutes per side.

7. Meanwhile, make the dip by adding all ingredients in a blender and puree them until smooth and creamy.

8. Once shrimps are golden brown, serve with mango dip and enjoy!

Nutrition: Calories 294,2, Fat 7, Carbs 31,2, Protein 26,6.

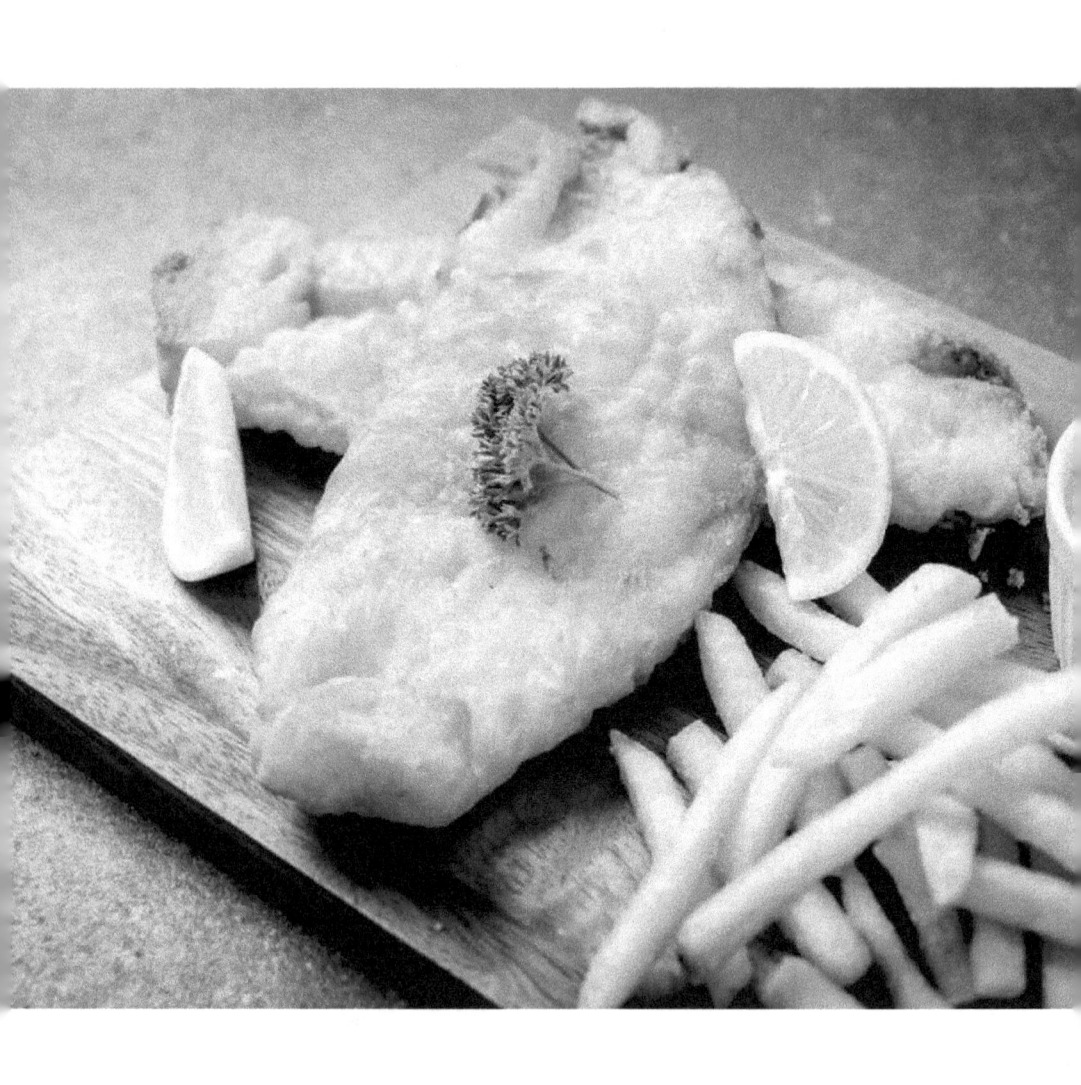

34. Crispy Fish

Preparation Time: 5 minutes

Cooking Time: 15 minutes

Servings: 4

Ingredients:
- Thick fish fillets
- ¼ cup all-purpose flour
- 1 egg
- 1 cup bread crumbs
- 2 tablespoons vegetables
- Lemon wedge

Directions:
1. In different dishes, add flour, egg, and breadcrumbs and set aside.
2. Dip each fish fillet first into the flour dish, then into the egg, and finally into bread crumbs.
3. Place each fish fillet in a heated skillet and cook for 4-5 minutes per side.
4. When it's ready, remove it from the pan and serve with lemon wedges.

Nutrition: Calories 189, Fat 17, Fiber 0, Carbs 2, Protein 7.

35. Cucumber-Basil Salsa on Halibut Pouches

Preparation Time: 10 minutes

Cooking Time: 17 minutes

Servings: 4

Ingredients:
- 1 lime, thinly sliced into 8 pieces
- 2 cups mustard greens, stems removed
- 2 teaspoon olive oil
- 4-5 radishes trimmed and quartered
- 4 4-oz skinless halibut filets
- 4 large fresh basil leaves
- Cayenne pepper to taste, optional
- Pepper and salt to taste

SALSA INGREDIENTS:
- 1 ½ cups diced cucumber
- 1 ½ finely chopped fresh basil leaves
- 2 teaspoon fresh lime juice
- Pepper and salt to taste

Directions:

1. Preheat the oven to 400°F and cut the parchment papers into four pieces of 15 x 12- inch rectangles. Lengthwise, fold in half and unfold pieces.
2. Season halibut fillets with pepper, salt, and cayenne.
3. Just to the right of the fold, place ½ cup of mustard greens, add a basil leaf on the center of mustard greens, and topped with one lime slice.
4. Around the greens make a layer of ¼ of the radishes, drizzle with ½ teaspoon of oil, and season with pepper and salt. Top it with a slice of halibut fillet.
5. Fold the parchment paper crimping the edges on beginning from one end to the other. Seal the end of the parchment paper pinch it.
6. Bake the pouches for about 15 to 17 minutes until halibut is flaky.
7. Meanwhile, make your salsa by mixing all salsa ingredients in a medium bowl.
8. Once halibut is cooked, remove it from the oven and make a tear on top, being very careful with the steam. Then, spoon ¼ of salsa per piece on top of halibut through the slit you have created. Serve and enjoy!

Nutrition: Calories 335,4, Fat 16,3, Carbs 22,1, Protein 20,2.

36. Curry Salmon with Mustard

Preparation Time: 10 minutes

Cooking Time: 8 minutes

Servings: 4

Ingredients:
- ¼ teaspoon ground red pepper or chili powder
- ¼ teaspoon ground turmeric
- ¼ teaspoon salt
- 1 teaspoon honey
- 1/8 teaspoon garlic powder or a minced garlic clove
- 2 teaspoons whole grain mustard
- 4 pcs. 6-oz salmon fillets

Directions:
1. Preheat the oven to broil and grease a baking dish with cooking spray.
2. In a small bowl, add salt, garlic powder, red pepper, turmeric, honey, and mustard, and mix well.
3. Place the salmon on the baking dish with the skin side down and spread evenly the mustard mixture on top of the salmon.
4. Broil the salmon for about 8 minutes until flaky. Then serve!

Nutrition: Calories 324, Fat 18,9, Carbs 2,9, Protein 34.

37. Dill Relish on White Sea Bass

Preparation Time: 10 minutes
Cooking Time: 12 minutes
Servings: 4
Ingredients:
- 1 ½ tablespoon chopped white onion
- 1 ½ teaspoon chopped fresh dill
- 1 lemon, quartered
- 1 teaspoon Dijon mustard
- 1 teaspoon lemon juice
- 1 teaspoon pickled baby capers, drained
- 4 pieces of 4-oz white sea bass fillets

Directions:
1. Preheat the oven to 375°F.
2. In a small bowl add lemon juice, mustard, dill, capers, and onions and mix well.
3. Prepare four aluminum foil squares, place 1 fillet per foil and squeeze a lemon wedge per fish.
4. Divide into 4 the dill spread and drizzle each fillet.
5. Close the foil over the fish securely and bake for about 12 minutes.

6. Remove from foil, transfer to a serving platter, serve, and enjoy.

Nutrition: Calories 115, Fat 1, Carbs 12, Protein 7.

38. Dijon Mustard and Lime Marinated Shrimp

Preparation Time: 10 minutes

Cooking Time: 10 minutes

Servings: 8

Ingredients:
- ½ cup fresh lime juice, and lime zest as garnish
- ½ cup of rice vinegar
- ½ teaspoon of hot sauce
- 1 bay leaf
- 1 cup of water
- 1 lb. uncooked shrimp, peeled and deveined
- 1 medium red onion, chopped
- 2 tablespoons of capers
- 2 tablespoons of Dijon mustard
- 3 whole cloves

Directions:
1. In a shallow baking dish mix hot sauce, mustard, capers, lime juice, and onion and set aside.
2. In a large saucepan add bay leaf, cloves, vinegar, and water and bring to a boil.

3. Once it boils, add shrimps and cook for a minute while stirring continuously.

4. Drain shrimps, pour them into onion mixture and refrigerate for 1 hour.

5. Serve shrimps cold and garnished with lime zest.

Nutrition: Calories 232,2, Fat 3, Carbs 15, Protein 17,8.

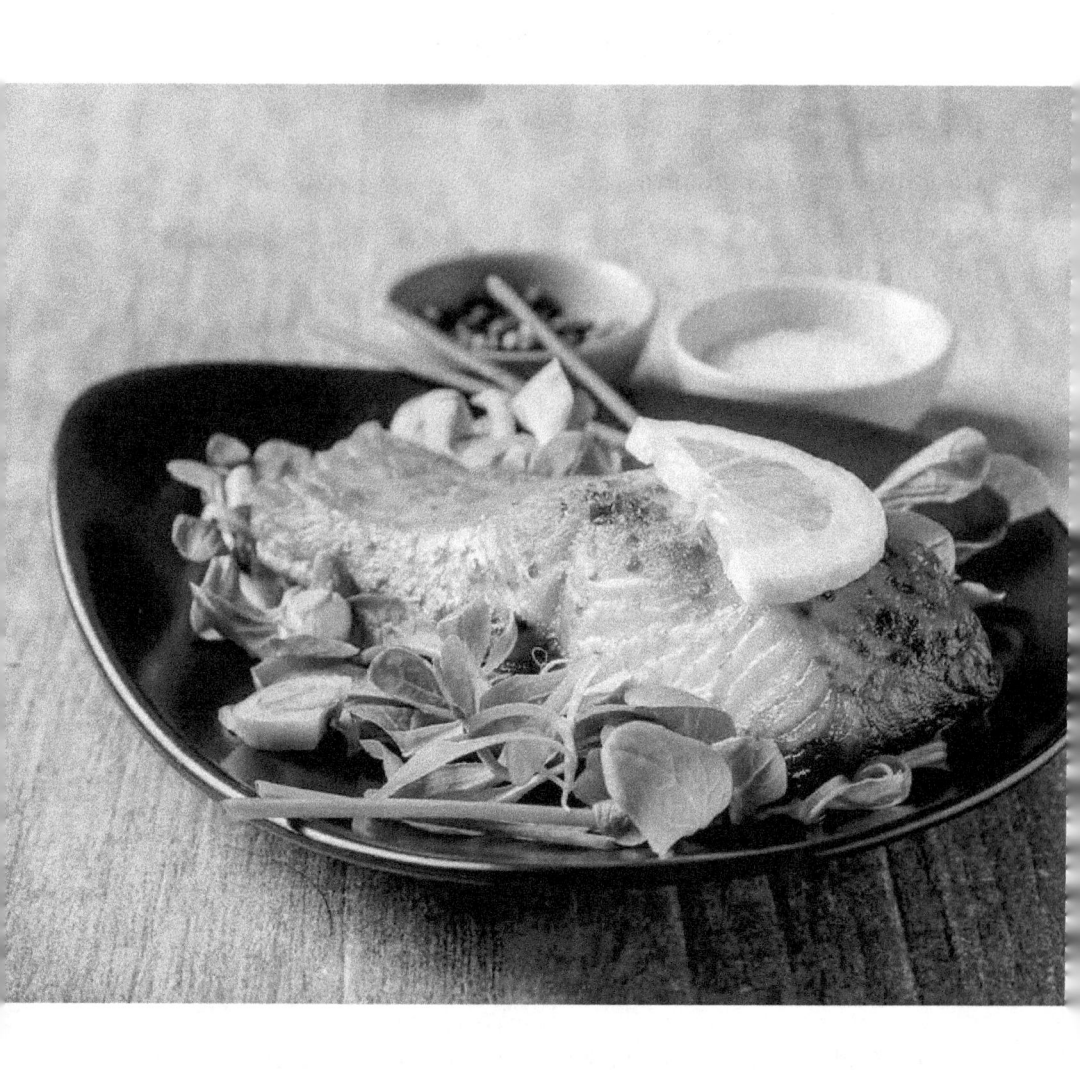

39. Healthy Salmon

Preparation Time: 10 minutes

Cooking Time: 10 minutes

Servings: 4

Ingredients:
- 1 tablespoon olive oil
- 1 small onion, diced
- ¼ cup chopped cilantro leaves and stems
- 1 to 2 chipotle peppers in adobo, diced
- 1/2 medium head of cauliflower, chopped
- 2 cups chicken broth (low sodium)
- 4 cups baby spinach
- 3/4 cup frozen corn
- 16 ounces Trifecta salmon
- 5-oz low-fat Greek yogurt
- Finishing salt
- Chili flakes

Directions:
1. In a large pot, heat oil, chopped onion, cilantro stems on med-high heat, and saute for about 3-4 minutes, until starting to brown.

2. Add chipotle peppers and cauliflower and cook for 1 to 2 minutes.

3. Add chicken broth and bring pot to a simmer, then lower the heat and cook for 5 minutes, or until cauliflower is tender.

4. Add spinach and corn and cook for 1 to 2 minutes.

5. Then, crumble the salmon to bite-size chunks and add to the pot reducing the heat to a gentle simmer.

6. At the end, remove from the heat, add Greek yogurt and stir.
7. Serve warm with finishing salt and chili flakes to taste!

40. Miso-Glazed Salmon

Preparation Time: 10 minutes

Cooking Time: 40 minutes

Servings: 4
Ingredients:
- ¼ cup red miso
- ¼ cup sake
- 1 tablespoon soy sauce
- 1 tablespoon vegetable oil
- 4 salmon fillets

Directions:
1. Into a bowl combine sake, oil, soy sauce, and miso and mix.
2. Rub mixture over salmon fillets and marinate them for 20-30 minutes in the fridge.
3. When the time is over, preheat a broiler and broil salmon for 5-10 minutes.
4. Serve and enjoy!

Nutrition: Calories 198, Fat 10, Fiber 2, Carbs 5, Protein 6.

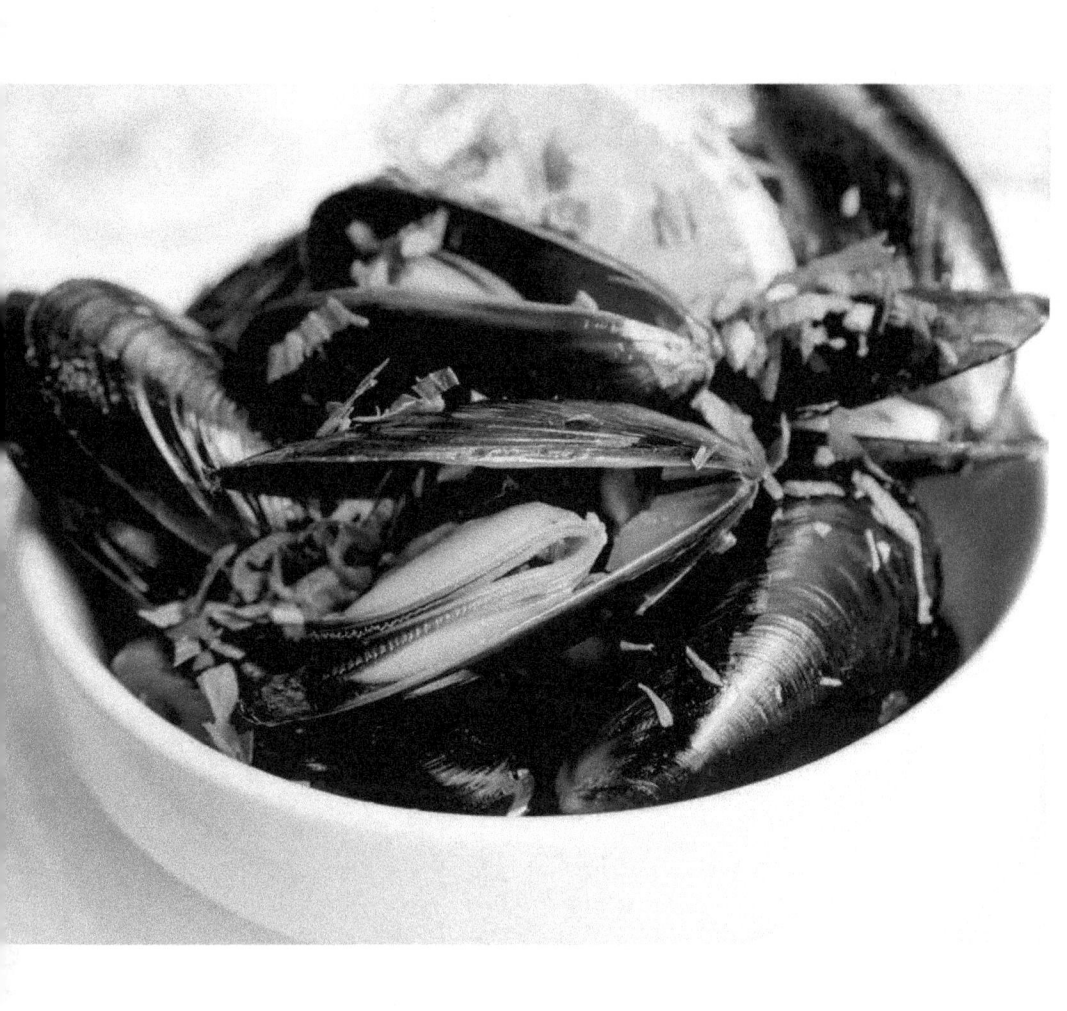

41. Mussels Mariners

Preparation Time: 10 minutes

Cooking Time: 30 minutes

Servings: 4

Ingredients:
- 2 tablespoons of unsalted butter
- 1 leek
- 1 shallot
- 2 cloves garlic
- 2 bay leaves
- 1 cup of white wine
- 2 lb. mussels
- 2 tablespoons of mayonnaise
- 1 tablespoon of lemon zest
- 2 tablespoons of parsley
- 1 sourdough bread

Directions:
1. In a saucepan melt butter, add leeks, garlic, bay leaves, and shallot, and cook until the vegetables are soft.
2. Bring to a boil, add mussels, and cook for 1-2 minutes.
3. Then, put the mussels aside and keep them warm

4. Meanwhile, whisk in the remaining butter with mayonnaise and then return mussels to the pot.

5. Add lemon juice, parsley lemon zest, and stir to combine.

6. Serve hot and enjoy.

Nutrition: Calories 321, Fat 17, Fiber 2, Carbs 2, Protein 9.

42. Salmon with Vegetables

Preparation Time: 10 minutes

Cooking Time: 15 minutes

Servings: 4

Ingredients:
- 2 tablespoons of olive oil
- 2 carrots
- 1 head fennel
- 2 squash
- ¼ onion
- 1-inch ginger
- 1 cup of white wine
- 2 cups of water
- 2 parsley sprigs
- 2 tarragon sprigs
- 6 oz. salmon fillets
- 1 cup of cherry tomatoes
- 1 scallion

Directions:
1. In a skillet heat olive oil, then add fennel, squash, onion, ginger, carrot, and cook until the vegetables are soft.

2. Add wine, water, parsley, and cook for another 4-5 minutes.
3. Meanwhile, season salmon fillets, then place them in the pan and cook them for 4-5 minutes per side or until is ready.
4. Serve the salmon into a bowl, accompanied by tomatoes and scallion around. Enjoy!

Nutrition: Calories 301, Fat 17, Fiber 4, Carbs 2, Protein 8.

43. Salmon Florentine

Preparation Time: 5 minutes

Cooking Time: 30 minutes

Servings: 4

Ingredients:
- 1 ½ cups of chopped cherry tomatoes
- ½ cup of chopped green onions
- 2 garlic cloves, minced
- 1 teaspoon of olive oil
- 1 quantity of 12 oz. package frozen chopped spinach, thawed and patted dry
- ¼ teaspoon of crushed red pepper flakes
- ½ cup of part-skim ricotta cheese
- ¼ teaspoon each for pepper and salt
- 4 quantities of 5 ½ oz. wild salmon fillets
- Cooking spray

Directions:
1. Preheat the oven to 350°F
2. In a skillet, heat the olive oil, then add the onions and cook them for about 2 minutes, until they become soft.

3. Add the spinach, red pepper flakes, tomatoes, pepper, and salt and cook for 2 minutes while stirring.

4. Remove the pan from the heat and let it cool for about 10 minutes.

5. When the vegetables have cooled down, stir in the ricotta and put a quarter of the spinach mixture on top of each salmon fillet.

6. Place the fillets on a lightly greased rimmed baking sheet and bake it for about 15 minutes.

7. When the salmon has been thoroughly cooked, serve, and enjoy!

Nutrition: Calories 350, Fat 13, Carbs 15, Protein 42.

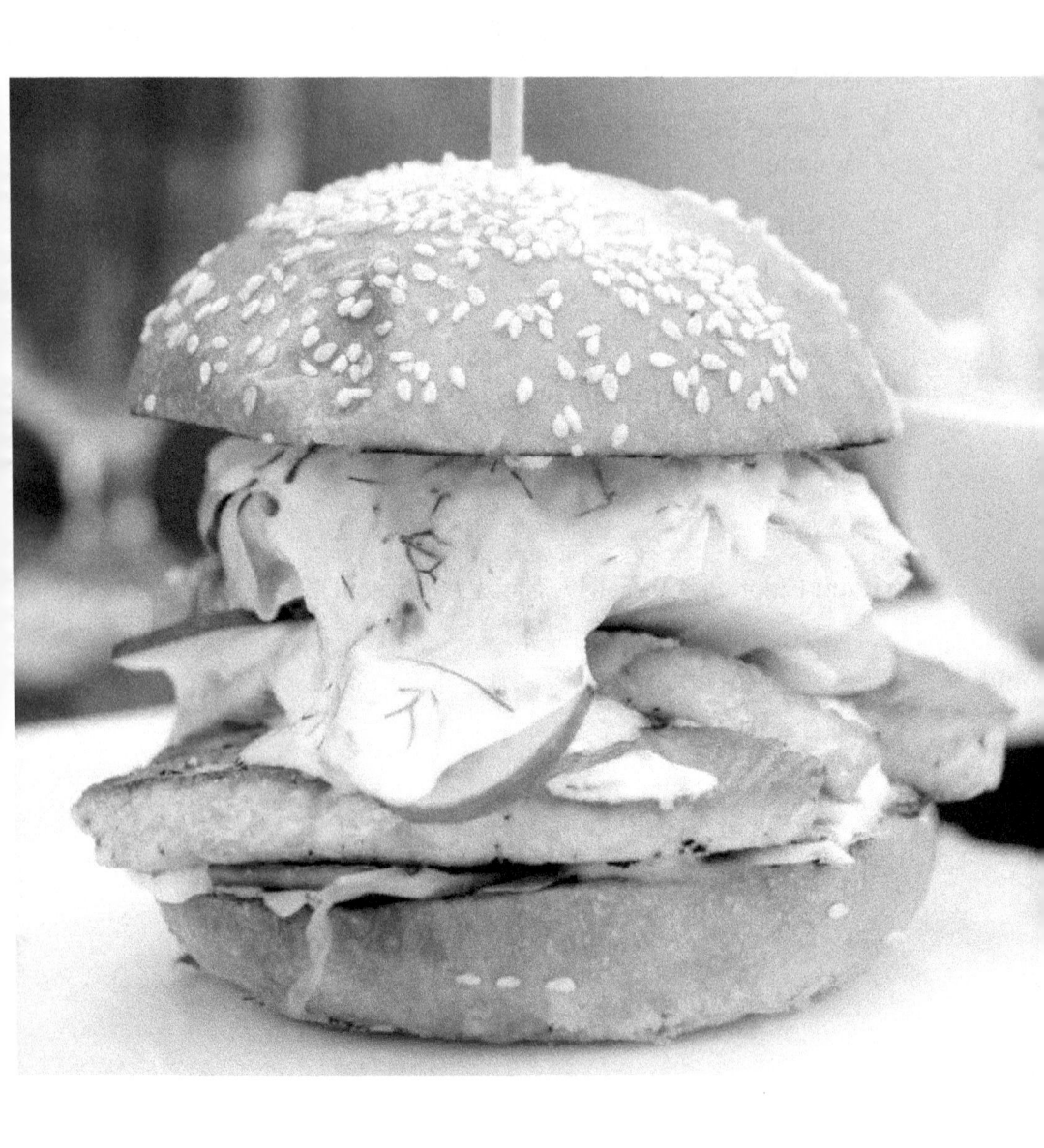

44. Salmon Burgers

Preparation Time: 10 minutes
Cooking Time: 15 minutes
Servings: 4
Ingredients:
- 1 lb. salmon fillets
- 1 onion
- ¼ dill fronds
- 1 tablespoon of honey
- 1 tablespoon horseradish
- 1 tablespoon of mustard
- 1 tablespoon olive oil
- 2 toasted split rolls
- 1 avocado

Directions:
1. Into a bowl, combine mustard, honey, mayonnaise, and dill.
2. Place salmon fillets in a blender and blend until smooth.
3. Transfer the smooth salmon to a bowl; add onion, dill, honey, horseradish, season with salt and pepper, mix well, and form 4 patties.
4. In a skillet, heat oil, add salmon patties, and cook for 2-3 minutes per side.

5. Meanwhile, divide lettuce and onion between the buns.

6. When salmon burgers are ready, remove them from heat and place the salmon patty on top of the buns.

7. Finish with a spoon of the mustard mixture on the top and avocado slices. Then serve and enjoy!

Nutrition: Calories 189, Fat 7, Fiber 4, Carbs 6, Protein 12.

45. Salmon Cakes

Preparation Time: 8 minutes

Cooking Time: 15 minutes

Servings: 4

Ingredients:
- 2/3 cup of panko bread crumbs
- 2 tbsp of canola mayonnaise
- 1 tbsp minced fresh parsley
- 2 tbsp chopped green onions
- 1 tsp dijon mustard
- ½ tsp Worcestershire sauce
- dash of salt
- dash of ground red pepper
- 1 large egg
- 8oz of trifecta salmon
- 1 tbsp of olive oil
- 1 lemon

Directions:
1. In a bowl, combine half of the panko bread crumbs and all of the ingredients up until the salmon.
2. Then, add in the salmon and mix well.
3. With your hands, shape the mixture into four patties.
4. Coat the patties with the remaining half of the panko bread crumbs.
5. In a griddle, add the olive oil and cook the salmon cakes for 3-4 minutes on each side or until they are golden brown.
6. Serve with broccoli and rice as a side.

46. Savory Cilantro Salmon

Preparation Time: 10 minutes

Cooking Time: 30 minutes

Servings: 4

Ingredients:
- 2 tablespoons of fresh lime or lemon
- 4 cups of fresh cilantro, divided
- 2 tablespoon of hot red pepper sauce
- ½ teaspoon of salt, divided
- 1 teaspoon of cumin
- 4,7 oz. of salmon filets
- ½ cup of (4 oz.) water
- 2 cups of sliced red bell pepper
- 2 cups of sliced yellow bell pepper
- 2 cups of sliced green bell pepper
- Cooking spray
- ½ teaspoon of pepper

Directions:
1. In a blender combine half of the cilantro, lime juice or lemon, cumin, hot red pepper sauce, water, and salt, then puree until they become smooth.

2. Transfer the marinade gotten into a large re-sealable plastic bag, add salmon to the marinade, and seal the bag, squeezing out the air that might have been trapped inside.

3. Turn to coat salmon and refrigerate for about one hour, turning as often as possible.

4. Preheat the oven to 400°F.

5. In a slightly-greased, medium-sized square baking dish, arrange the pepper slices in a single layer and bake it for 20 minutes, turning the pepper slices sometimes.

6. Remove the salmon from the marinade and drain it.

7. Crust the upper part of the salmon with the remaining chopped, fresh cilantro, then place salmon on top of the pepper slices and bake for about 12-14 minutes.

8. Remove from the oven and serve!

Nutrition: Calories 350, Fat 13, Carbs 15, Protein 42.

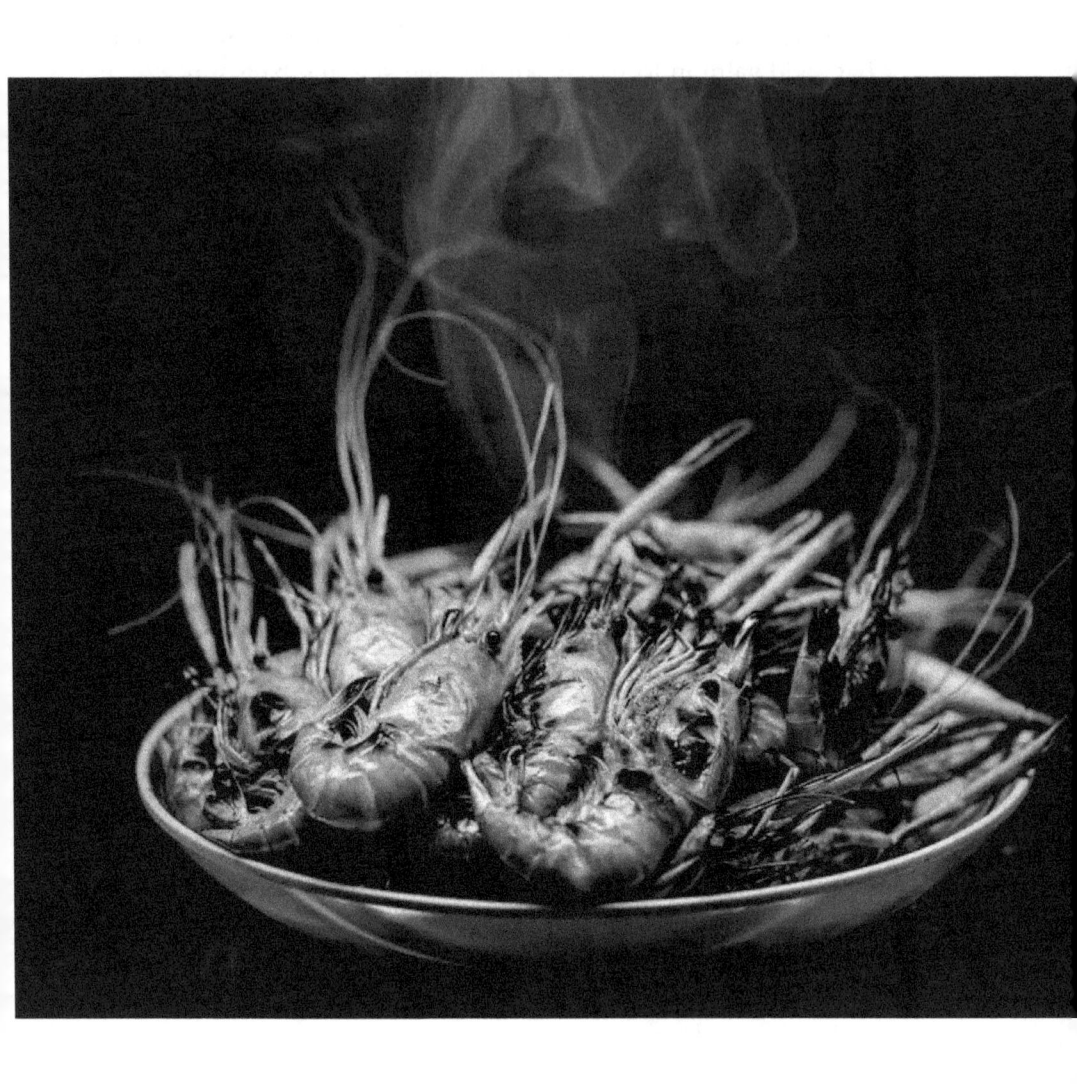

47. Scampi Grilled Shrimp

Preparation Time: 15 minutes

Cooking Time: 20 minutes

Servings: 4

Ingredients:
- 1 ¾ lb of wild-caught large shrimp, shells removed
- 4 teaspoons of lemon or roasted garlic oil
- ½ tablespoon of seasoning (or use a mixture of lemon, garlic, parsley, onion, lime, salt)

Directions:
1. Add all the ingredients into a bowl and allow it to settle.
2. Meanwhile, preheat the grill to medium-high heat and place the seasoned shrimp on it.
3. Cook for about 20 minutes (or until it turns dark pink), stirring occasionally.
4. Serve and enjoy!

Nutrition: Calories 242, Fat 7,4, Fiber 0, Carbs 2,6, Protein 38,7.

48. Seared Scallops

Preparation Time: 15 minutes

Cooking Time: 20 minutes

Servings: 4

Ingredients:
- 1 lb. sea scallops
- 1 tablespoon of canola oil

Directions:
1. Season scallops and let them rest in the fridge for a few minutes.
2. In a skillet, heat oil, add scallops, and cook them for 1-2 minutes per side.
3. When they're ready, remove them from heat and serve. Enjoy!

Nutrition: Calories 283, Fat 8, Fiber 2, Carbs 10, Protein 9.

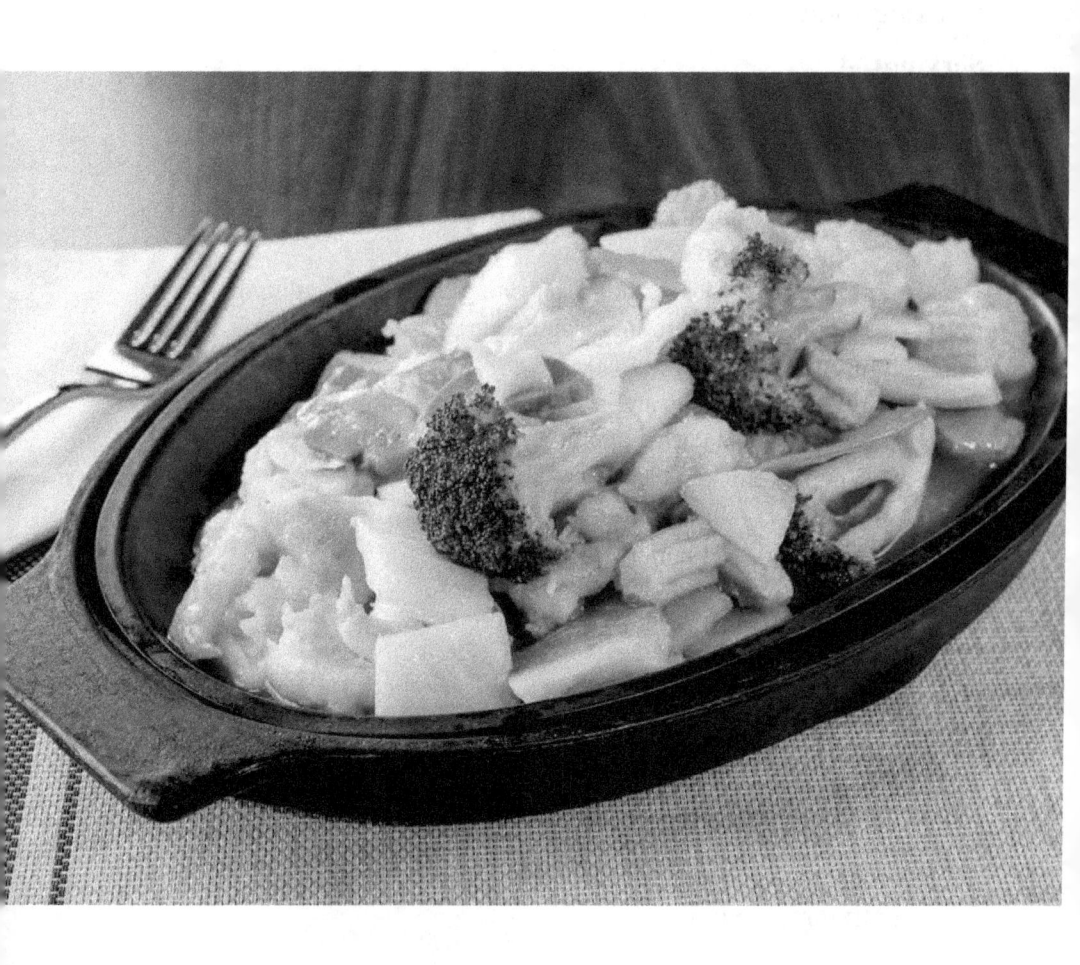

49. Shrimp Broccoli

Preparation Time: 15 minutes

Cooking Time: 10 minutes

Servings: 4

Ingredients:
- 4 teaspoons of roasted garlic oil (you can use fresh garlic or any other oil you like)
- 1 ¾ lb of shrimp (wild-caught, thawed with shells removed)
- 2 cup of fresh broccoli florets
- 2 teaspoon of rockin' ranch seasoning (or use a mixture of tarragon, chives, lemon, black pepper, garlic, salt, parsley, and onion)
- 1 teaspoon of garlic and spring onion seasoning (or use a mixture of lemon, fresh garlic, and onion)
- 1/3 cup of chicken broth (low sodium)
- 4 cups of noodles of choice (like hearts of palm noodles)
- 2 tablespoons of butter

Directions:
1. Add the oil to a pan and heat up over medium-high heat.
2. Add the shrimp and cook for about 1minute on each side.
3. Add the broth and seasonings and stir gently.
4. Add the broccoli, cover the pan with the lid, and bring the mixture to a boil.
5. When it boils, reduce heat to medium and cook for about 2 min, or until the broccoli turns bright green.
6. Add the butter, stir, and add the noodles.

7. Once the mixture becomes very hot serve and enjoy!

Nutrition: Calories 340, Fat 12, Fiber 3,3, Carbs 12,4, Protein 45,7.

50. Shrimp Chives Chipotle

Preparation Time: 5 minutes

Cooking Time: 15 minutes

Servings: 4

Ingredients:
- 4 teaspoons of roasted garlic oil (or use any other oil and fresh garlic)
- 1 cup of chives (or scallions greens; chopped)
- 2 lbs of raw shrimp (wild-caught, shelled, and deveined with tails completely removed)
- 1 can (about 16 oz) unflavored and no sugar added tomatoes (diced)
- 1 tablespoon of cinnamon chipotle (or use a small amount of cinnamon, chipotle pepper, salt, and pepper)
- 4 lime wedges
- 4 tablespoons of fresh cilantro

Directions:
1. Add the oil to a pan and heat over medium-high heat.
2. Then, add scallion and cook for 1 minute, or until it becomes wilted.
3. Add the shrimp and cook for 1 minute on each side.
4. Add the cinnamon seasoning and tomatoes, and cook for another 5 minutes or until the shrimp is fully cooked stirring occasionally.
5. Serve sprinkling over with the cilantro and lime wedges. Enjoy!

Nutrition: Calories 250, Fat 3,6, Fiber 1,5, Carbs 6,2, Protein 46,1.

51. Shrimp Curry

Preparation Time: 15 minutes

Cooking Time: 20 minutes

Servings: 4

Ingredients:
- 2 tablespoons of peanut oil
- ¼ onion
- 2 cloves garlic
- 1 teaspoon ginger
- 1 teaspoon cumin
- 1 teaspoon turmeric
- 1 teaspoon paprika
- ¼ red chili powder
- 1 can tomatoes
- 1 can coconut milk
- 1 lb. peeled shrimp
- 1 tablespoon cilantro

Directions:
1. In a skillet, add onion and cook for 4-5 minutes.
2. Add ginger, cumin, garlic, chili, and paprika, and cook on low heat for a few minutes.

3. Pour the tomatoes and the coconut milk and simmer for 10-12 minutes.

4. Add in shrimp and cilantro, and cook them for 2-3 minutes stirring slowly.

5. Serve and enjoy!

Nutrition: Calories 178, Fat 17, Carbs 3, Protein 9.

CPSIA information can be obtained
at www.ICGtesting.com
Printed in the USA
BVHW080226190521
607644BV00013B/1309